Exercise Testing and Prescription Lab Manual

Second Edition

Edmund O. Acevedo, PhD, FACSM

Health and Human Performance
Virginia Commonwealth University

Michael A. Starks, PhD, CSCS

College of Counseling, Educational Psychology, and Research
The University of Memphis

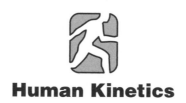

Human Kinetics

Library of Congress Cataloging-in-Publication Data

Acevedo, Edmund O.

   Exercise testing and prescription lab manual / Edmund O. Acevedo, Michael A. Starks. -- 2nd ed.

       p. cm.

  Includes bibliographical references.

  ISBN-13: 978-0-97360-8728-5 (soft cover)

  ISBN-10: 0-7360-8728-1 (soft cover)

  1. Exercise tests--Laboratory manuals. 2. Exercise therapy--Laboratory manuals. I. Starks, Michael A. II. Title.

  RC683.5.E94A24 2011

  615.8'2--dc22

2010048662

ISBN-10: 0-7360-8728-1 (print)

ISBN-13: 978-0-7360-8728-5 (print)

Copyright © 2011, 2003 by Edmund O. Acevedo and Michael A. Starks

The Web addresses cited in this text were current as of September 2010, unless otherwise noted.

Acquisitions Editor: Loarn D. Robertson, PhD; **Developmental Editor:** Judy Park; **Assistant Editor:** Brendan Shea; **Copyeditor:** Joanna Hatzopoulos Portman; **Permission Manager:** Dalene Reeder; **Graphic Designer:** Joe Buck; **Graphic Artist:** Denise Lowry; **Cover Designer:** Keith Blomberg; **Photographer (cover):** Human Kinetics; **Photographs (interior):** Courtesy of Edmund O. Acevedo. Photo on page 10 © Human Kinetics. Photo on page 153 courtesy of Michael A. Starks; **Photo Asset Manager:** Laura Fitch; **Visual Production Assistant:** Joyce Brumfield; **Photo Production Manager:** Jason Allen; **Art Manager:** Kelly Hendren; **Associate Art Manager:** Alan L. Wilborn; **Illustrations:** © Human Kinetics; **Printer:** United Graphics

Printed in the United States of America   10 9 8 7 6

The paper in this book is certified under a sustainable forestry program.

Human Kinetics
Web site: www.HumanKinetics.com

United States: Human Kinetics, P.O. Box 5076, Champaign, IL 61825-5076
800-747-4457
e-mail: humank@hkusa.com

Canada: Human Kinetics, 475 Devonshire Road Unit 100, Windsor, ON N8Y 2L5
800-465-7301 (in Canada only)
e-mail: info@hkcanada.com

Europe: Human Kinetics, 107 Bradford Road, Stanningley, Leeds LS28 6AT, United Kingdom
+44 (0) 113 255 5665
e-mail: hk@hkeurope.com

Australia: Human Kinetics, 57A Price Avenue, Lower Mitcham, South Australia 5062
08 8372 0999
e-mail: info@hkaustralia.com

New Zealand: Human Kinetics, P.O. Box 80, Torrens Park, South Australia 5062
0800 222 062
e-mail: info@hknewzealand.com

E4980

To my wonderful wife and best friend, Tracy
and my children, Eddie and Elena

—EOA

Contents

List of Tables

Preface

The health benefits of regular physical activity are unquestionable. Furthermore, researchers have defined exercise guidelines that clarify the safest, most effective, and most efficient manner of physical activity participation. The American College of Sports Medicine (ACSM) has established the gold standard for professional practice and certification in exercise testing and prescription. ACSM was the first organization to certify health and fitness professionals and, since 1975, has certified more than 45,000 professionals in 44 countries. The Health Fitness Specialist (HFS) certification has had the greatest number of participants. This laboratory manual addresses the necessary skills and techniques for successful completion of the HFS certification.

A HFS certified professional is qualified to assess, design, and implement fitness programs for apparently healthy individuals and for individuals with controlled disease. Certification guidelines are presented in *ACSM's Guidelines for Exercise Testing and Prescription, Eighth Edition*. A component of the requirements for each certification, including HFS, is a practical application of the knowledge and skills associated with exercise testing and prescription. This *Exercise Testing and Prescription Lab Manual* is an excellent supplement to undergraduate courses that prepare students to take the ACSM HFS certification examination. The experiential learning labs are easy to follow and correspond with the practical skills required for successful completion of the HFS certification exam.

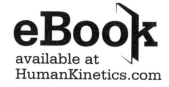

How This Lab Manual Is Organized

Similar to the first edition, this lab manual contains three sections: part I, Pretest Responsibilities; part II, Techniques in Exercise Testing; and part III, Exercise Prescription. The first section includes three labs that focus on the HFS's responsibilities before performing an exercise test. These labs address safety procedures, requirements for exercise testing equipment, calibration of equipment, medical history evaluation, risk factor evaluation and stratification, and informed consent. This edition includes instructions for calibration of laboratory instruments and 10 new case studies that highlight a breadth of examples that represent a hypokinetic population. Case studies direct significant attention toward risk factor evaluation and stratification.

The second section includes seven labs that focus on the techniques used in assessing the components of health-related fitness (cardiorespiratory, body composition, muscular strength and endurance, and flexibility). To allow for more concentrated attention on skill development in assessing HR and BP, this edition has separate labs for assessing HR and BP and for assessing skinfold thickness and circumferences. The application procedures in these labs include step-by-step instructions, data collection worksheets, diagrams depicting appropriate techniques, and charts that present norms for comparisons within an individual's age and sex category.

The final section of this manual focuses on exercise prescription. In this edition the metabolic calculations in the first lab (lab 11) include an answer key. The next two labs (labs 12 and 13) address the three phases of exercise prescription (initial, improvement, and maintenance) and the assessment of a participant's goals and commitment to the physical activity prescription. The final lab (lab 14) challenges students to apply the techniques and principles presented in the manual through the development of case studies.

The appendixes provide a summary of the effects of common pharmacological agents on cardiorespiratory responses at rest, common metric conversions used in exercise testing and prescription calculations, and a list of metabolic and anthropometric formulas.

Practical Learning Features

Each lab features an easy to follow format including the headings Purpose, Materials, Background Information, Procedures, Discussion Questions, and References or Bibliography. The Background Information section provides a framework for the lab but does not necessarily present all the knowledge required for an understanding of the rationale, theory, and physiological principles of the topics presented in that lab. We expect that more in-depth knowledge will be presented in a course lecture format or that students will research topics further to be able to answer discussion questions they do not understand. The Procedures section contains the steps required to complete the lab. Many labs require data collection. To facilitate this process, this manual contains all the forms and worksheets necessary to complete the lab assignments and collect the data in an organized manner. These forms and worksheets are located in appendixes A and B and owners of this manual may photocopy them. Each lab identifies how many copies of which forms are needed to complete it so that students can bring enough copies of the appropriate forms and worksheets to that lab. Once the students who have purchased the manual become practitioners, they may also copy forms from appendixes A and B for use with their clients. A glossary defines terms appearing in the text and appendixes.

New to This Edition

This second edition addresses the updates necessary to be consistent with the recent modifications that ACSM has published (*ACSM's Guidelines for Exercise Testing and Prescription, Eighth Edition*). This edition also includes added background and rationale in the introduction of a number of chapters, in particular, information that addresses the importance of the assessment and how the assessment relates to overall program development. Finally, this edition's enhanced discussion questions will appropriately challenge students by incorporating greater analysis of the information provided in the corresponding lab.

In response to student feedback about the first edition, the organization of this manual has been changed slightly to focus on taking the reader through each progressive phase of exercise testing and prescription. In addition, students will find enhanced instructions for skills and techniques that are critical for preparing for the HFS certification exam. The progression of labs through the testing and prescription process, the easy to follow instructions, and the practical worksheets make this lab manual the perfect experiential component for a course in exercise testing and prescription. It is a wonderful tool for individuals who have taken the challenge of preparing themselves for the HFS certification.

This manual takes the reader through each progressive phase of exercise testing and prescription. These practical experiences are intended to coincide with a lecture course that presents the required knowledge base for HFS certification.

This manual fills a void for the health fitness practitioner studying for the HFS certification exam with a focused presentation of the skills included in the exam. Each lab is presented in a way that can be easily followed independent of additional instruction. Furthermore, each lab has worksheets that facilitate the practical experience. The labs match directly with the practical skills evaluated on the HFS exam and thus provide an excellent tool for facilitating preparation.

Acknowledgments

This second edition lab manual has evolved in parallel with contemporary standards for the application of exercise testing techniques and physical activity prescription. A number of colleagues have provided critical feedback that has influenced the improvements made to this manual. We would like to acknowledge those individuals:

Drs. Michael Meyers and Robert Kraemer provided valuable input and critical review of the labs. The work of Terry Garner, Naomi Howard, and Jason VanGotten, who were also completing their graduate assistantship responsibilities, greatly enhanced the presentation of the labs. Finally, the first author would like to express his appreciation to his wife, Tracy Acevedo, for her heartfelt support and her editorial expertise.

PART

I

Pretest Responsibilities

Part I comprises three labs that focus on the HFS's responsibilities before performing an exercise test. These labs present information pertaining to safety procedures, requirements for exercise testing equipment, calibration of equipment, medical history evaluation, risk factor evaluation and stratification, and informed consent. Case studies direct significant attention toward risk factor evaluation and stratification.

Orientation to Lab Instruments, Procedures, and Responsibilities

Purpose

This lab familiarizes students with the safety procedures, lab equipment, and instruments that they will use during labs throughout the course. It explains the procedures, requirements, and responsibilities for lab assignments.

Materials

- Cycle ergometer (e.g., Monark, Tunturi)
- 12-lead electrocardiograph (ECG) (electrodes and cables)
- 3-lead ECG telemetry system (electrodes and transmitters)
- Treadmill
- Rating of perceived exertion (RPE) scale
- Flexibility assessment devices (e.g., goniometer, sit-and-reach box, meter stick or yardstick)
- Mercurial and aneroid sphygmomanometer
- Stethoscope
- Hand dynamometer
- Barometer and thermometer
- Scale and stadiometer
- Body composition assessment devices

Procedures

1. The lab instructor describes preliminary preparation for exercise testing. The following elements are crucial to a safe, professional exercise testing environment and the fitness specialist should be familiar with them.

    a. Establishing emergency procedures

    b. Periodically practicing emergency drills

    c. Clearly posting emergency phone numbers

    d. Ensuring current CPR certification

    e. Maintaining an appropriately professional (clean, quiet, visually appealing) environment for testing

    f. Establishing policies to ensure adequate client privacy

    g. Checking and calibrating equipment frequently

2. The lab instructor discusses the procedures and grading system.

3. The lab instructor briefly introduces and describes the items listed under Materials. Students will practice using this equipment as they participate in the labs that follow in this course.

4. Review the units of the metric system (appendix D).

5. Discuss the general lab instructions below that should be followed for each lab.

General Laboratory Instructions

1. Before each scheduled lab, read the instructions to become familiar with the materials you will use and the procedure you will follow.

2. The lab instructor will give additional verbal clarification and demonstrations when necessary. Listen and take notes as applicable.

3. You will usually work in groups of three or four. Organize your group quickly, selecting a recorder, a subject, and a technician. Become familiar with the responsibilities that each position entails. If data are to be collected from more than one subject, rotate assignments during each lab. (Note: Obtain data from all group members when possible.)

4. One member of the group should be responsible for obtaining the equipment needed for the day, maintaining it accordingly during the work period, and returning it after the lab period. Be extremely careful with all equipment; it is very expensive and difficult to replace. Return all equipment to the exact place from which it was taken, make sure it is clean, and keep the storage facility well organized.

5. The recorder should record the observations immediately as they are taken. Record only raw data; perform any calculations and conversions after the data are collected.

6. Work seriously and quietly. Noise may disrupt the subject or interfere with accurate reporting of the results. If basal rates are to be established or if blood pressures are to be recorded, eliminate all noise.

7. Listen to final instructions. Do not leave the lab before checking with the lab instructor.

8. Appropriate clothing (shorts, T-shirt, sweats, athletic shoes, and socks) is required. In addition, you will need a calculator for computing data.

9. Complete lab assignments, including discussion questions, after each lab meeting. Type the labs and hand them in before the next scheduled lab begins.

Calibrating Lab Instruments

Purpose

This lab demonstrates how to calibrate equipment for exercise testing and prescription and why such calibration is important.

Materials

- Cycle ergometer
- Sphygmomanometer
- Weight scale
- Hanging scale
- One copy of the Cycle Ergometer Calibration Worksheet (appendix B, page 118)
- One copy of the Sphygmomanometer Calibration Worksheet (appendix B, page 119)
- One copy of the Weight Scale Calibration Worksheet (appendix B, page 120)
- One copy of the Hanging Scale Calibration Worksheet (appendix B, page 121)

Background Information

When inaccurate instruments are used in a procedure, they introduce error. The process of adjusting or correcting an instrument to coincide with a known standard is called *calibration*. Calibration is essential to obtaining reliable and valid data. In the simplest case, two scales of measurement might be compared with each other. For example, if we lay a meter stick alongside some reference measure, we can then compare the lengths and subdivisions of the two. In this case, to correct any error we might have to sand off the existing markings on the meter stick and etch new ones along the entire scale.

A reference quantity previously determined to be within an acceptably small degree of error can be used as a calibration standard (reference measure). For example, a set of brass weight standards might be used to calibrate a balance scale for accurate weighing. In the case of a sophisticated electronic balance, adjustments can be made to reconcile small deviations of measurement from known weights. Some instruments, however, have no simple means of adjustment.

Error

Two kinds of measurement errors exist: random errors and systematic errors. **Random errors** occur in all measurement, but good technique and consistency of methods can minimize them. You can estimate the degree of random error by performing repeated measurements on the same quantity with the same instrument and expressing the variability of the measurement with some statistic (i.e., standard error). **Systematic errors** arise when an instrument or procedure consistently overestimates or underestimates the quantities being measured.

The errors estimated in laboratory work are generally random errors. If a systematic error is detected, adjust the instrument (or procedure) to eliminate it.

Calibration Points

Consider the calibration of a hand dynamometer, which measures the strength of a person's handgrip. To check it for accuracy, you might secure its base to a supporting framework and suspend 50 kg of mass from its stirrup. Under these conditions, the pointer should be aligned with the 50 kg readout display. This procedure, however, would establish only whether the dial correctly indicates the acceleration of gravity on a mass of 50 kg. To be certain of the accuracy of the instrument throughout the range of its scale readings, you would need to check every distinguishable point within this range. Such a procedure is not generally practical. A reasonable compromise is to check several calibration points centered at about the middle of the expected range as well as several points at about the lowest and highest expected measurements. If the relationship between the actual and measured values for a quantity is consistent in a rigorous (mathematical) manner, then it may be sufficient to calibrate an instrument at only a few points.

Linearity

Linearity is the maximum percentage of error between the expected value and the actual reading, throughout an instrument's measurement range. If the numerical values of the calibration points and the numerical values of the readings obtained with an instrument lie in a straight line when they are graphed, the instrument is said to be *linear*. Most instruments are nearly linear only over a certain range of values, and the manufacturer often specifies this range. If a reasonably linear response can be assumed for an instrument, it is necessary to calibrate it only at two points and assume that all other measurements lie on the line through these points. In actual practice, because instruments are not perfectly linear, and because measurements are seldom exactly reproducible, a line of best fit is often drawn to describe data points from the readings of an instrument as compared with the actual values of the calibration standards. The graphs in figure 2.1 depict various examples of lines and curves that could be present when calibrating exercise testing equipment. The x-axis represents five standards that increase an equal amount from one measurement to the next. The y-axis presents the measure taken by the instrument that is being calibrated. Figure 2.1a depicts a positive linear relationship, which means that as one measure increases, the other measure also increases to the same degree. Figure 2.1b depicts a negative relationship, which indicates that as one variable increases, the other decreases. Figure 2.1c depicts a curvilinear relationship, which indicates that the device you are calibrating measures accurately only within a specific range (e.g., skinfold calipers often are not accurate beyond a specific range). Figure 2.1*d* depicts varying points whose relationship can best be represented with a line of best fit. Not every point will fit on the line. Very sensitive instruments often require the use of a line of best fit.

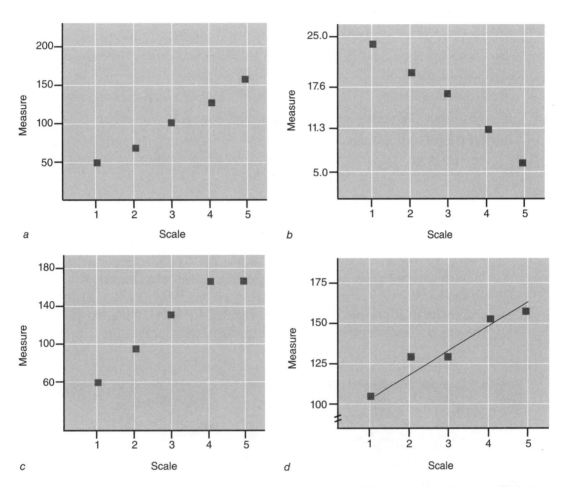

Figure 2.1 Examples of lines and curves that could be present when calibrating exercise-testing equipment: a positive linear relationship *(a)*, a negative relationship *(b)*, a curvilinear relationship *(c)*, and varying points whose relationship can most accurately be represented with a line of best fit *(d)*.

Procedures

1. Follow the instructions for calibrating the following equipment.
2. Complete the worksheets provided for each instrument.

Cycle Ergometer

This procedure applies to the steps for calibrating the belt resistance on a belt-braked bike (e.g., Monark, Tunturi). Note that both ends of the belt that passes around the rim of the wheels are attached to a revolving drum to which a pendulum is fixed. Thus, the device acts as a pendulum scale, measuring the difference in tractive efforts (resistance slowing down the wheel) at the two ends of the belt. The belt can be stretched with the lever that is adjusted with the handwheel. The deflection of the pendulum is read on a scale graduated in kiloponds (kp; equal to a kilogram) and Newtons (N). The braking power (kp) multiplied by the distance pedaled gives the amount of work in kilopond meters (kpm).

1. Be sure the bike is sitting on a level surface.
2. Remove the forward attachment of the belt from the pendulum.
3. Attach at least two different known calibration weights to the pendulum and read the scale.
4. Record the reading of the measured weights displayed on the scale (figure 2.2).
5. If the scale does not read accurately, calibration will be required.
6. With a person sitting on the bike without feet touching the pedals, change the zero mark on the scale with the calibration gauge adjustor so that it coincides with the mark on the pendulum weight.
7. Attach a known weight to the pendulum and read the scale. Record the reading of the measured weights displayed on the scale.
8. Check the linearity by hanging at least two different weights and recording the scale readings.
9. Graph the results of both measures by plotting the actual resistance of the known calibration weights (x-axis) against the scale readings (y-axis) on the **Cycle Ergometer Calibration Worksheet** provided for this calibration procedure. The graph should represent a positive linear relationship (figure 2.1*a*, page 9).

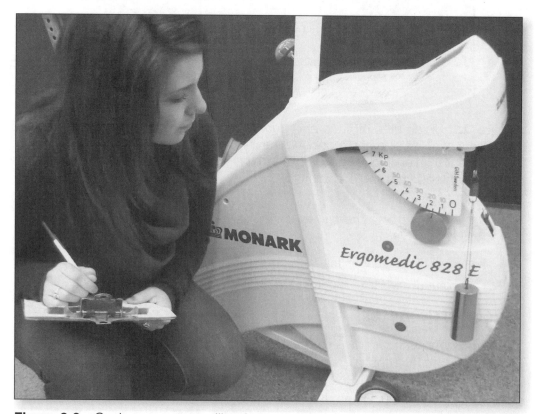

Figure 2.2   Cycle ergometer calibration.

Sphygmomanometer

A **sphygmomanometer** is a blood pressure measurement system composed of an inflatable rubber bladder, an instrument to indicate applied pressure, an inflation bulb to create pressure, and an adjustment valve to deflate the system. Of these, the cuff and the pressure-measuring instrument are the most crucial to the accuracy of the measurement (Perloff et al. 1993). To ensure accurate measurements, you must use the appropriate cuff size. When inflated the bladder should encircle at least 80% of the upper arm and not cause a bulging or displacement. If the bladder is too wide, blood pressure will be underestimated; if too narrow, pressure will be overestimated. Consequently, bladder sizes vary for children (arm girth 13-20 cm; 8 cm wide by 13 cm long), adults (arm girth 24-32 cm; 13 cm wide by 24 cm long), and large adults (arm girth 32-42 cm; 17 cm wide by 32 cm long).

The pressure-measuring device can be of the mercury or aneroid type (ACSM 2010). The mercury type is the standard. Its calibration is easily maintained. The mercury column should rise and fall smoothly, form a clear meniscus, and read zero when the bladder is deflated. If sticking occurs, clean the inside of the column according to the specific manufacturer's recommendations. If mercury falls below zero, add mercury. The mercurial sphygmomanometer should be read at the top of the mercury bubble as the level falls. The aneroid gauge uses a metal bellows assembly that expands when pressure is applied. When the bladder is deflated, a spring moves the attached pointer to zero. This gauge should be calibrated once every 6 months at a variety of settings using a mercury column. A simple Y tube is used to connect the two systems together. Take readings with pressure falling to simulate the readings during an actual measurement. If the aneroid gauge is not in calibration, return it to the manufacturer for calibration, or dispose of it and replace it.

1. Check to be sure that both gauges, one from the mercury column and one from the aneroid gauge, are set to zero.
2. Inflate the cuff to a pressure that reads 200 mmHg on the mercury column.
3. Record this reading and the reading from the aneroid gauge on the **Sphygmomanometer Calibration Worksheet** provided for this calibration procedure.
4. Repeat procedures 1 through 3 for the following inflation pressures: 180 mmHg, 160 mmHg, 140 mmHg, 120 mmHg, 100 mmHg, 80 mmHg, 60 mmHg, and 40 mmHg.
5. Graph the results of both measures by plotting the pressure readings from the mercury column against the aneroid gauge on the **Sphygmomonometer Calibration Worksheet**.

Scale

A scale is a measuring instrument used to determine the gross weight of an object. The instrument can be digital, as in the case of a hanging scale; spring resistance, as in a Chatillon scale; or a balance beam scale (commonly found in a physician's office). Maintain the accuracy of the instruments through daily assessment and calibration. After the instruments have been calibrated, you can use a set of known weight standards to verify the calibration. The weights can be either suspended from the device or placed on the platform, depending on the instrument. When verifying the calibration, use at least two different known weights.

The digital scale, or hanging scale, usually has a self-calibration system that is found within the device or a calibration button that resets the scale to zero. To calibrate this type of scale, either turn the device off and back on or press the reset button. Graph the results by plotting the weights against the scale readings on the **Weight Scale Calibration Worksheet** provided for this procedure.

The **Chatillon scale**, a type of hanging scale, measures weight through pressure resistance on an internal spring system. This type of scale has an adjustment screw or knob that can be turned to calibrate the unweighted device display to zero. Graph the results by plotting the weights against the scale readings on the **Hanging Scale Calibration Worksheet** provided for this procedure.

The balance beam scale, often referred to as a *physician's scale,* has an adjustment screw on the end of the balance beam. With the scale unweighted and the slide weights set at zero, turn the adjustment screw until the beam arm is centered, indicating that the device is zeroed. Graph the results by plotting the weights against the scale readings on the **Weight Scale Calibration Worksheet** provided for this procedure.

Discussion Questions

1. Why is calibration important?
2. Describe and give examples of sources of random error and systematic error.
3. What does lack of linearity suggest about the accuracy of a lab instrument or technique?
4. Describe what a line of best fit represents.
5. Did the instruments tested require calibration? Please explain either a yes or no answer.

References

ACSM (American College of Sports Medicine). 2010. *ACSM's guidelines for exercise testing and prescription.* 8th ed. Baltimore: Lippincott Williams & Wilkins.

Perloff, D., C. Grim, J. Flack, E.D. Frohlich, M. Hill, M. MacDonald, and B.Z. Morgenstern. 1993. Human blood pressure determination by sphygmomanometry. *Circulation* 88: 2460-2470.

Risk Factor Evaluation, Medical History, and Informed Consent

Purpose

This lab presents the appropriate procedures and specific content necessary for gaining the client's informed consent. This lab includes case studies in which you will be required to evaluate the client's risk factors and place him or her in the appropriate classification.

Materials

- *ACSM's Guidelines for Exercise Testing and Prescription, Eighth Edition,* chapters 1, 2, 3
- One copy of the Medical History Form (appendix A, page 102) or the Health Screening Form (appendix A, page 105)
- One copy of the Informed Consent Form (appendix A, page 106)
- One copy of the Physician Release Form (appendix A, page 107)
- Ten copies of the Risk Stratification Form (appendix A, page 108)

Background Information

Risk stratification was developed for exercise professionals in an attempt to improve safety and reduce risk of injury for clients before they undergo exercise testing and physical activity. Risk stratification is based on known factors that may predict cardiovascular disease such as age, family history, previous and current health status, medical history, and current activity levels (Howley and Franks 2007). From this information the exercise professional can classify an individual into one of three categories. The American College of Sports Medicine (2010) has developed tables that allow the exercise professional to best decide on the appropriate classification category for each individual client. This classification category gives guidance to the exercise professional on whether a physician should be present and what type of exercise regimen should be followed.

Before evaluating the 10 case studies, become familiar with tables 3.1 through 3.3 on pages 14 through 15. Through years of clinical research and professional experience, ACSM has developed these guidelines and recommendations. The ACSM's Initial Risk Stratification table (3.1) allows fitness professionals to categorize individuals according to risk factors and signs or symptoms to aid in triage and other decision-making processes. The recommendations in table 3.2 provide general guidance on the need for a medical examination and exercise testing before participation in a moderate-to-vigorous exercise program, and physician supervision of exercise.

Table 3.1 ACSM's Initial Risk Stratification

Low risk	Asymptomatic men and women who have ≤1 CVD risk factor from table 3.3
Moderate risk	Asymptomatic men and women who have ≥2 risk factors from table 3.3

High risk	Individuals with
	• known cardiac, peripheral vascular, or cerebrovascular disease; chronic obstructive pulmonary disease, asthma, interstitial lung disease, or cystic fibrosis; or diabetes mellitus (type 1 and 2), thyroid disorders, renal or liver disease; or
	• one or more of the following signs or symptoms:
	  - heart murmur;
	  - unexplained fatigue;
	  - dizziness or fainting;
	  - swelling of the ankles;
	  - fast or irregular heartbeat;
	  - unexplained shortness of breath;
	  - intermittent lameness or pain in calf muscles;
	  - breathing discomfort when not in upright position, or interrupted breathing at night; or
	  - pain or discomfort in the jaw, neck, chest, arms, or elsewhere that could be caused by lack of circulation.

Adapted from American College of Sports Medicine 2010.

When studying table 3.2, it is important to note that **moderate exercise** is defined as activities that are approximately 3 to 6 metabolic equivalents (METs) or the equivalent of brisk walking at 3 to 4 mph for most healthy adults. Nevertheless, some sedentary or older persons might consider a pace of 3 to 4 mph to be "hard" to "very hard." Moderate exercise may alternatively be defined as an intensity well within the client's capacity, one that the client can comfortably sustain for a prolonged period (about 45 min), has a gradual initiation and progression, and is generally noncompetitive. If a person's exercise capacity is known, relative moderate exercise may be defined by the range 40 to 60% of maximal oxygen uptake. **Vigorous exercise** is defined as activities of greater that 6 METs or, alternatively, an exercise intense enough to represent a substantial cardiorespiratory challenge. If a person's exercise capacity is known, vigorous exercise may be defined as an intensity of greater than 60% maximum oxygen uptake.

Table 3.2 ACSM's Recommendations

	Low risk	Moderate risk	High risk
Current (within past year) medical examination and exercise testing before participation			
Moderate exercise	Not necessary[1]	Not necessary	Recommended[2]
Vigorous exercise	Not necessary	Recommended	Recommended
Physician supervision of exercise tests			
Submaximal test	Not necessary	Not necessary	Recommended
Maximal test	Not necessary	Recommended	Recommended

[1]The designation *not necessary* reflects that a medical examination, exercise test, and physician supervision of the exercise test are not essential in the preparticipation screening but should not be viewed as inappropriate.

[2]When physician supervision of exercise testing is *recommended,* the physician should be readily available in close proximity should an emergent need develop.

Adapted from American College of Sports Medicine 2010.

Table 3.3 Atherosclerotic Cardiovascular Disease (CVD) Risk Factor Thresholds for Use With ACSM Risk Stratification

Positive risk factors	Defining criteria
Age	Men ≥45 yr; Women ≥55 yr
Family history	Myocardial infarction, coronary revascularization, or sudden death before 55 yr of age in father or other male first-degree relative (i.e., brother or son), or before 65 yr of age in mother or other female first-degree relative (i.e., sister or daughter)
Cigarette smoking	Current cigarette smoker or person who quit within the previous 6 mo or had exposure to environmental tobacco smoke
Sedentary lifestyle	Not participating in a regular exercise program or meeting the minimal physical activity recommendations[†] of the CDC and from the U.S. Surgeon General's report
Obesity[‡]	Body mass index is ≥30 kg/m², or waist girth is >102 cm (40 in.) for men and >88 cm (35 in.) for women
Hypertension	Systolic blood pressure is ≥140 mmHg or diastolic is ≥90 mmHg, confirmed by measurements on at least 2 separate occasions, or on antihypertensive medication
Dyslipidemia	Low-density lipoprotein (LDL-C) cholesterol is ≥130 mg/dL (3.37 mmol/L) or high-density lipoprotein (HDL-C) cholesterol is <40 mg/dL (1.04 mmol/L) or on lipid-lowering medication. If total serum cholesterol is all that is available use ≥200 mg/dL (5.18 mmol/L)
Impaired fasting glucose	Fasting blood glucose is ≥100 mg/dL (5.5 mmol/L) but <126 mg/dL (6.93 mmol/L), confirmed by measurements on at least 2 separate occasions
Negative risk factor	**Defining criteria**
High-serum HDL cholesterol[§]	>60 mg/dL (1.55 mmol/L)

[†]Accumulating 30 minutes or more of moderate physical activity on most days of the week.

[‡]Professional opinions vary regarding the most appropriate markers and thresholds for obesity, therefore allied health professionals should use clinical judgment when evaluating this risk factor.

[§]It is common to sum risk factors in making clinical judgments. If HDL is high, subtract one risk factor from the sum of positive risk factors, because high HDL decreases CVD risk.

Adapted from American College of Sports Medicine 2010.

Table 3.3 presents the risk factor thresholds used to determine if an individual meets the criteria for a positive risk. The number of positive risk factors is summed. However, because of the cardioprotective effect of high-density lipoprotein cholesterol (HDL-C), for individuals with HDL-C that is ≥60 mg/dL, one positive risk factor is subtracted from the total number of positive risk factors.

You will note a great deal of variation in the medical histories and case studies. Throughout your career, the information you will have available or will be able to obtain on clients will also vary widely. By dealing with the range of styles and levels of information completeness presented in these case studies, you will become more proficient at reading different types of reports and assessing the pertinent information for the purpose of risk stratification.

Procedures

1. The lab instructor gives a short lecture on risk factor evaluation and informed consent.
2. The lab instructor explains the use of the following forms:
   a. **Medical History Form** and **Health Screening Form**, which can be used if a shorter form is desired
   b. **Informed Consent Form**
   c. **Physician Release Form**
   d. **Risk Stratification Form**
3. The lab instructor presents case studies 1 through 10 (pages 17-26).
4. Complete or answer the following for each of the 10 case studies.
   a. Complete a **Risk Stratification Form** for each case study.
   b. Would you recommend a medical examination and exercise testing before the client begins moderate exercise? Vigorous exercise?
   c. Would you recommend physician supervision of a submaximal exercise test? Maximal exercise test?
   d. What are some other areas of concern you may need to address? Does this client require referral for further health or nutritional counseling?

Discussion Questions

1. To give valid consent to a procedure, what characteristics must a client maintain?
2. What are the seven components of a valid informed consent procedure and form?
3. What should be included in a medical history evaluation?
4. What are the components of the physical exam and the laboratory tests?

References

ACSM (American College of Sports Medicine). 2010. *ACSM's guidelines for exercise testing and prescription*. 8th ed. Baltimore: Lippincott Williams & Wilkins.

Howley, E.T., and B.D. Franks. 2007. *Fitness professional's handbook*. 5th ed. Champaign, IL: Human Kinetics.

Case Study 1

Demography

Age: 24
Ht: 5 ft 2 in. (157.5 cm)
Sex: Female
Race: Black
Wt: 112 lb (50.9 kg)

Family History

Father (age 67) had a quadruple bypass at the age of 46. Mother (age 57) had two transient ischemic attacks this year. Older brother (age 35) had stints implanted for coronary artery blockage.

Medical History

Present Conditions

A recent physical exam revealed no health concerns. This client has a resting heart rate (HR) of 58 beats per minute (bpm) and her resting blood pressure (BP) in 108/68. She has a total cholesterol of 198 mg/dL. Her high-density lipoprotein (HDL) level is 65 mg/dL and triglycerides are 110 mg/dL. She recently had a maximal oxygen consumption test that indicates her $\dot{V}O_2$max is 51 ml/kg/min. The electrocardiogram (ECG) results of the maximal stress test indicated no known abnormalities.

Past Conditions

This client has reported no past medical problems.

Behavior and Risk Assessment

The client reports she likes to exercise 1.5 to 2 hours per day. She works out in the gym weight training 45 minutes and runs on the treadmill for 45 minutes to an hour each exercise session. She runs 3 miles a day, 5 days a week to and from her job as a nurse. She has a diet that consists of lean sources of protein and is rich in complex carbohydrate and vegetables. The client states she is obsessed with staying healthy due to her immediate family's health conditions.

Case Study 2

Demography

Age: 48
Ht: 5 ft 11 in. (180.3 cm)
Sex: Male
Race: Hispanic
Wt: 189 lb (85.9 kg)

Family History

Father (age 73) and mother (age 71) are both living and are very active and healthy. Both parents participate in 5 K races on a regular basis. Three siblings (ages 30, 44, and 46) are also very active and healthy.

Medical History

Present Conditions

This client recently had a complete physical with blood analysis. Examination revealed the following information about this client:

Resting HR: 46   **Resting BP:** 112/70
Total cholesterol: 180 mg/dL   **HDL cholesterol:** 75 mg/dL
Triglycerides: 90 mg/dL   **Body fat:** 16%
Fasting blood glucose: 83 mg/dL $\dot{V}O_2$**max:** 52.5 ml/kg/min
ECG: Left ventricular hypertrophy

Past Conditions

This client reports no past medical problems

Behavior and Risk Assessment

The client is planning on competing in the Iron Man Hawaii later this year. He currently runs between 35 and 70 miles per week depending on the time of year. He has been an avid runner for over 25 years but has never been a swimmer or cyclist.

Case Study 3

Demography

Age: 30
Ht: 5 ft 7 in. (170.2 cm)
Sex: Male
Race: White
Wt: 247 lb (112.3 kg)

Family History

His father died from heart disease at age 63. His mother is still alive at age 75. He has no siblings.

Medical History

Present Conditions

This client has no personal history of coronary heart disease. His blood lipid profile indicates a total cholesterol value of 223 mg/dL, HDL cholesterol of 34mg/dL, triglycerides of 132 mg/dl, and blood glucose of 110 mg/dl. Two years ago, the client's resting blood pressure was measured at 161/99, he was put on a loop diuretic, and today his resting blood pressure is 120/78. A resting electrocardiogram reveals normal rate and rhythm. The client reports no history of chest pain, but has noticed some shortness of breath lately when climbing stairs.

Past Conditions

The client had surgery for carpel tunnel syndrome three years ago. No other conditions are reported.

Behavior and Risk Assessment

The client is a former smoker who quit 6 months ago. He also likes to drink a highball after work before dinner each night. The subject does not perform regular aerobic exercise but circuit trains with weights 3 days a week. His current body fat level has been measured at 32%. He recently had a maximal $\dot{V}O_2$ test performed and the results indicate his maximal MET level to be 7.

Case Study 4

Demography

Age: 36

Ht: 5 ft 6 in. (167.6 cm)

Sex: Female

Race: Asian American

Wt: 127 lb (57.7 kg)

Family History

Father (age 66) and mother (age 64) are both living, active, and healthy. Two siblings (ages 31 and 32) are also both very active and healthy.

Medical History

Present Conditions

This client's blood lipid profile revealed a total cholesterol of 148 mg/dL, HDL of 71 mg/dL, triglycerides of 68 mg/dL, and blood glucose of 89 mg/dL. Resting blood pressure was measured at 118/70. The resting ECG reveals a resting heart rate of 48 beats per minute with probable left ventricular hypertrophy. She reported occasional heart palpitations but the ECG indicated no abnormalities. Her current body fat level is 12.4%.

Past Conditions

This client reports she had surgery for bone spurs in her right calcaneous two years ago and has been symptom free since.

Behavior and Risk Assessment

The subject works as a purchasing agent for a large retail chain. She drinks 2 to 3 cups of coffee in the morning before leaving for work. Breakfast usually consist of a granola bar and an energy drink. She typically eats a microwave dinner for lunch and usually only takes 30 minutes or less on her lunch break. She compensates for the short lunch break by eating an energy bar and drinking an energy drink on her breaks. Dinner usually consists of a salad and soup. She only drinks alcohol occasionally at family functions. She participates in a local Pilates class at the YWCA 3 nights a week and runs 2 to 3 miles a day.

Case Study 5

Demography

Age: 43
Ht: 6 ft (182.9 cm)
Sex: Male
Race: White
Wt: 224 lb (101.8 kg)

Family History

This client's mother died from heart disease at age 63. His father is still alive at the age 69. The client has a younger sibling, age 32, who is apparently healthy and active.

Medical History

Present Conditions

The client has noticed considerable lack of energy and incentive to exercise. His friend has encouraged him to join a local basketball league geared toward middle-aged adults. He has recently been examined by his physician to determine the suitability of an exercise program for him. He has a maximal MET level of 7. Health screening tests indicate the following information:

Resting HR: 98   **Resting BP:** 128/86
Total cholesterol: 210 mg/dL   **HDL Cholesterol:** 61 mg/dL
Triglycerides: 158 mg/dL   **Fasting blood glucose:** 100 mg/dL
Body Fat: 32%

Past Conditions

This client played basketball at a small private college. During his senior year he broke his right ankle playing the final game. He has reported no complications or problems from the injury since.

Behavior and Risk Assessment

The client has never smoked and only drinks alcohol once or twice a week. His job requires that he travel at least 2 days a week. He does not exercise regularly and would like to get back into the shape he was in 22 years ago, when he was in college. The client is not currently participating in any structured exercise program.

Case Study 6

Demography

Age: 27
Ht: 5 ft 10 in. (177.8 cm)
Sex: Male
Race: Black
Wt: 238 lb (108.2 kg)

Family History

The client's mother died from complications as a result of type 2 diabetes at the age of 52. His father died from prostate cancer at 37. His 47-year-old sister recently underwent a double bypass surgery for blocked coronary arteries.

Medical History

Present Conditions

The client has not had a physical exam in 5 years. Blood analysis and vital statistics were obtained at a community health fair. The client's blood cholesterol was measured at 268 mg/dL, with and HDL value of 29 mg/dL. Triglycerides were 232 mg/dL, while his blood glucose level was 145 mg/dL. Liver enzymes in the blood were greatly elevated. Blood uric and creatinine levels were also elevated. His resting blood pressure is 166/90 and resting heart rate is 92 bpm.

Past Conditions

The client self-disclosed he was underweight as a small child and has had difficulty gaining weight in the past.

Behavior and Risk Assessment

The subject is a state-level amateur bodybuilder. He recently won a local national qualifying competition in his weight division and wants to go on to the junior national championships. In an attempt to increase his lean mass and decrease body fat levels to ensure success he has begun taking black market steroids without medical supervision. He has noticed a marked increase in his lean mass and decrease in body fat percentage but is bothered by the increased acne. He eats a diet that consists primarily of lean chicken, fish, and egg whites along with small quantities of vegetables. He does aerobic training 20 minutes a day by walking at 3 mph. He drinks only distilled water.

Case Study 7

Demography

Age: 26
Ht: 5 ft 5 in. (165.1 cm)
Sex: Female
Race: White
Wt: 185 lb (84.1 kg)

Family History

This client's father died at age 44 from a myocardial infarction. Her mother is still alive at 58 with no cardiovascular problems. She has an older sister age 39 and a younger brother age 25. Neither has had any reported cardiovascular or other health related problems.

Medical History

Present Conditions

The client has a resting heart rate of 89 bpm. Her resting blood pressure is 144/94. A fasting blood lipid profile revealed total cholesterol of 243 mg/dL, HDL cholesterol of 22 mg/dL, triglycerides of 212 mg/dL, and a blood glucose value of 245 mg/dL.

Past Conditions

The client has not had a physical exam in 2 years. The exam 2 years ago revealed multiple premature atrial contractions. The client chose not to seek further medical attention against the advice of her physician. The stress test performed during the exam indicated the client had a maximum MET level of 4.5.

Behavior and Risk Assessment

The client reports being a heavy chain smoker of at least three packs of cigarettes per day. The subject also drinks a minimum of 6 cups of coffee every night while working at an answering service. She reports that she eats primarily drive-through fast food for the convenience. She drinks 4 to 6 alcoholic beverages nightly. The only physical activity she participates in is playing billiards at the local pool hall.

Case Study 8

Demography

Age: 32

Ht: 5 ft 7 in. (170.2 cm)

Sex: Female

Race: Native American

Wt: 118 lb (53.6 kg)

Family History

This client's father (age 75) and mother (age 73) are in excellent health and have no known medical conditions. She has an older brother (age 38), a younger brother (age 31), and a younger sister (age 28). All her siblings are in good health and have no apparent medical conditions.

Medical History

Present Conditions

The client has noticed a major decrease in her energy level. She has recently been examined by her physician to determine the cause of her lethargic feelings. She has a maximal MET level of 12. Health screening tests indicate the following information:

Resting HR: 53	**Resting BP:** 110/68
Total cholesterol: 160 mg/dL	**HDL Cholesterol:** 68 mg/dL
Triglycerides: 60 mg/dL	**Fasting blood glucose:** 85 mg/dL
Body Fat: 16%	

The physical exam revealed the client also had a low blood iron level of 40 μg/dL. Other than these findings the client is apparently healthy.

Past Conditions

This client has only had one medical concern when she was 15 years old. She fractured her left foot as a result of stepping in a hole during a high school cross country race. She has had no reported medical problems since. The client had a previous maximal MET level of 13.5.

Behavior and Risk Assessment

This client currently competes in triathlons, road races, and running events. She has competed every weekend for the past two years. She currently logs a minimum of 30 miles per week running, 50 miles per week cycling, and swimming at least 10 miles per week. She has not taken a break from this training regimen for 5 years. Her personal times in the competitive events have started to decline. To compensate for the poor performances she is contemplating whether she needs to increase her training volume.

Case Study 9

Demography

Age: 61
Ht: 5 ft 6 in. (167.6 cm)
Sex: Male
Race: Asian American
Wt: 155 lb (70.5 kg)

Family History

This client's mother had a heart attack at age 62 and underwent a 3-vessel coronary bypass graft surgery at the age of 63. His father died of a heart attack at the age of 42. He has two brothers, one age 58, and one age 53, who are both alive and healthy.

Medical History

Present Conditions

The physical exam revealed a highly fit Asian American male. The client's blood pressure at the time of the exam was 116/60 with a regular pulse of 48 bpm. The client had a normal ECG readout. His orthopedic exam revealed good flexibility and minor limitations on the left shoulder. All the client's extremities showed good pulses. He has been in generally good physical condition all his life. At age 27 he was diagnosed to be hypertensive. His blood pressure at rest was 142/90 and during stressful situations could increase to as high as 176/110. At age 27 he began taking a diuretic to maintain his blood pressure at 120/80. At age 30 his medication was changed to a beta blocker. His blood pressure while on this medication has stabilized at 112/66. He has no restrictions placed on him at this time. This subject eats no pork or fried foods and uses no caffeine products. His present cholesterol level is 195 mg/dL and triglycerides are 38 mg/dL.

Past Conditions

In the past the client has had several bouts of ischemia. The client had rotator cuff surgery performed on his left shoulder at the age of 44 and still experiences an occasional recurrence of pain.

Behavior and Risk Assessment

This client has never smoked. He drinks 3 to 6 oz of sake on the weekend, but never drinks any alcoholic beverages during the week. He eats a small breakfast, a light lunch, and a moderate size dinner of primarily vegetables, chicken or fish. He does, however, salt his food heavily. He sleeps 7 or 8 hours a night. This individual averages 12 hours a day at his job running an international import/export business. This client jogs 3 miles, 5 days a week before work. He also exercises on a game system for 20 minutes, 3 days a week, in his office at noon. He presently has a body composition of 12.7% body fat and has lost approximately 25 pounds in the last 2 years. He has a functional MET level of 12.

Case Study 10

Demography

Age: 54

Ht: 5 ft 8 in. (172.7 cm)

Sex: Female

Race: Hispanic

Wt: 127 lb (57.7 kg)

Family History

This client's father died at age 44 from influenza. Her mother died at age 53 from pneumonia. She has an older brother age 56 who is still alive that recently had two stints implanted for coronary blockage.

Medical History

Present Conditions

A recent physical exam revealed that at night she has cramping in her lower legs accompanied by increased perspiration. This client recently had a blood lipid profile that revealed a total cholesterol of 210 mg/dL, HDL cholesterol of 45 mg/dL, triglycerides of 200 mg/dl, and blood glucose of 105 mg/dl. She reports occasional palpitations in her chest during the morning, but has no chest pain or personal history of heart problems. A recent graded stress test indicated negative for any cardiac abnormalities. The stress test also measured her $\dot{V}O_2$max at 24.5 ml/kg/min.

Past Conditions

The client reports a history of anxiety-related disorders due to the loss of her parents at an early age. She takes anti-anxiety medication, which she states is helping her cope with the losses.

Behavior and Risk Assessment

The subject works as a real estate agent in a large metropolitan city. She drinks 2 cups of coffee each morning. Breakfast usually consists of a microwave breakfast burrito or a meal from a fast food restaurant. She typically eats at a fast food restaurant for lunch and she usually only takes 30 minutes or less at her lunch break. She compensates for the short lunch breaks by eating a fast food meal between real estate showings. She consumes approximately 2 to 4 alcohol drinks nightly with prospective clients or coworkers. Dinner usually consists of a reduced-calorie microwave meal. She is sedentary, but wishes to begin an exercise program to look and feel better. She has never smoked, but some of the workers in her office are moderate smokers.

PART

II

Techniques in Exercise Testing

Part II comprises seven labs that focus on the techniques used to assess the components of health-related fitness (cardiorespiratory function, muscular strength and endurance, flexibility, and body composition), including information on ECG placement and operating ECG equipment. The application procedures in these labs include step-by-step instructions, diagrams depicting appropriate techniques, and charts that present norms for making comparisons by age and gender. Forms for recording data are in appendix A. Because many of these forms will be used more than once during the course, make photocopies before using them.

Heart Rate and Blood Pressure Assessment Techniques

Purpose

This lab introduces the specific measurement techniques for assessing heart rate (HR) and blood pressure (BP).

Materials

- Stopwatch
- Stethoscope
- Sphygmomanometer
- Cycle ergometer
- One copy of the Heart Rate and Blood Pressure Data Collection Worksheet (appendix B, page 123)

Background Information

Familiarity with assessment tools and techniques is essential to accurate exercise testing. Through repeated practice with the devices and guidance from a qualified instructor, you can develop the skills necessary to accurately test and measure the specific variables and become proficient in exercise testing.

When assessing components of health-related fitness (cardiorespiratory function, muscular strength and endurance, flexibility, and body composition) you must understand two concepts: reliability and validity.

Reliability is the extent to which your assessment yields the same result on repeated trials. In fitness testing, we are primarily concerned with test-retest reliability and interrater reliability. Test–retest reliability addresses the consistency of your fitness assessment over time (i.e., your ability to accurately assess BP today, tomorrow, and next week). Interrater reliability determines the consistency of one tester's assessment with that of another tester. When learning to perform a fitness assessment, your assessment will likely be compared with that of another person, possibly the instructor, to assess the accuracy of your assessment.

Validity refers to the accuracy of your assessment. It addresses whether or not you are assessing what you have intended to assess. In general, validity is determined by comparing your fitness assessment with another measure that is referred to as a *criterion measure*. For example, we can compare your body composition calculations taken with skinfold calipers to body composition assessment through hydrostatic weighing. Reliability (consistency) of an assessment can be very good, and yet your assessment may not be accurate (valid). Validity of an assessment is essential.

Monitoring HR and BP is the easiest and quickest method of assessing an individual's health and exercise status. To ensure that these and other test results are reliable and valid, always address the following factors:

Environmental factors can impact the reliability and validity of a fitness test. The testing room or laboratory should be a comfortable, clean environment with adequate lighting, good ventilation, and controlled temperature and humidity. A temperature range of 22 °C (71.6 °F) to 26 °C (78.8 °F) with adequate air movement is considered comfortable for exercise. Because cardiovascular responses can become variable when humidity exceeds 60%, a cool, dry environment (50% humidity) is recommended to dissipate the body heat produced during exercise.

When performing fitness tests it is also important to address the client's preparedness for the task. The client should be well rested and prepared for physical activity. To reduce the possibility of an anxiety response, provide a clear explanation of the all procedures and maintain a professional, relaxed atmosphere.

Heart Rate Technique

HR and work intensity are linearly related—that is, one increases proportionately with the other. When you measure HR, you can determine how hard the body is working and how it is responding to exercise. HR is a physiological parameter that is easy to monitor. However, because HR can be affected by numerous pharmacological agents it is important to identify the medications that a participant is taking and determine whether or not medication is affecting HR or BP. Appendix C contains a list of pharmacological agents and their effects on cardiorespiratory responses to exercise.

You can monitor HR by palpating a superficial artery, a procedure that is universally known as *taking the pulse*. During exercise, the most common site for monitoring HR is the radial artery, which descends on the lateral (thumb) side of the forearm to become quite superficial at the distal end of the radius. Taking the pulse at this end consists of compressing the artery against the anterior surface of the distal end of the radius (see figure 4.1). You can also find a pulse in the temporal artery, brachial artery, femoral artery, popliteal artery, posterior tibial artery, and dorsalis pedis artery.

The common carotid arteries on both sides of the neck have anatomic landmarks that are similar to each other. The common carotid pulse in the neck is bounded by the body of the mandible (lower jaw), the sternocleidomastoid muscle, and the larynx (i.e., Adam's apple). Palpate the carotid arterial pulses by gently compressing inward and backward along the anterior border of the sternocleidomastoid muscle at the level of the thyroid cartilage.

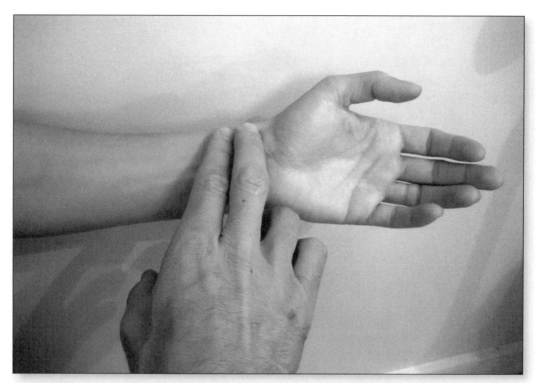

Figure 4.1 Taking the radial pulse.

Palpate the carotid pulses singly (one carotid artery at a time) by placing the first two fingers (not the thumb) lightly on the artery. Reports have shown that palpitation of the carotid artery after exercise has ended may produce bradycardia in some people. In addition, this method is inappropriate for participants who have various forms of vascular disease that affects the sensitivity of the carotid sinus.

Blood Pressure Technique

When you monitor BP, you can determine whether the cardiovascular system is adapting properly to the exercise or is posing undue stress on the body. BP is an important indicator of cardiorespiratory function at rest, during physical work, and during emotional stress.

When measuring BP, wrap the blood pressure cuff snugly around the person's upper arm, locating the center of the cuff bladder over the brachial artery and the bottom of the cuff 1 in. above the antecubital fossa (fold in the arm), as shown in figure 4.2. Tighten the valve on the bulb and begin to inflate. Place the head of the stethoscope on the brachial artery (located between the midline and the medial portion of the antecubital space). Inflate the cuff to the point at which the pulse disappears, then add an additional 20 to 30 mmHg (200 mmHg). The 200 mmHg will be read from the mercury column or the aneroid scale. This represents the amount of pressure required to raise a column of mercury 200 mm. Begin deflating immediately at a rate of 2 to 3 mmHg/sec. Record the first sound heard as the systolic BP (Korotkoff phase I), or the pressure exerted against the walls of the arteries during heart muscle contraction. The disappearance of sound (Korotkoff phase V) is considered the diastolic BP, or the pressure exerted against the artery walls during the relaxation phase of the contraction. A normal BP reading is 120/80 mmHg; 120 reflects the systolic pressure and 80

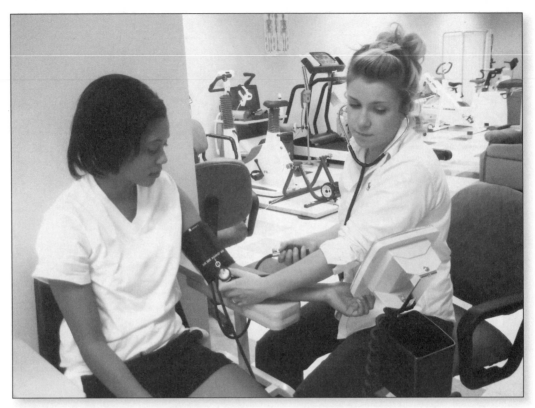

Figure 4.2 Location of the blood pressure cuff, with the center over the brachial artery and the bottom of the cuff 1 in. above the anetcubital fossa.

reflects the diastolic pressure. As you release the valve to deflate the cuff, watch the meter to match the sound changes with the numbers on the gauge. If you have no idea what the normal range is for the person you are testing, it is appropriate to ask. This information will decrease the risk of overinflation that may be uncomfortable.

Procedures

1. In groups of three to five, practice taking HR and BP on each other. Record your own resting HR and BP on the **Heart Rate and Blood Pressure Data Collection Worksheet.**

2. After obtaining resting data, have one person from each group exercise on a cycle ergometer for 12 min (four 3-min stages). The cyclist will maintain a pedaling rate of 50 rpm for the duration of the exercise. After 2 or 3 min of unloaded warm-up, increase the resistance to 0.5 kg during the first stage. Increase each subsequent stage by 0.5 kg (e.g., 0.5 to 1.0 kg, to 1.5 kg).

3. Monitor HR and BP during the 12 min of exercise and 3 min of recovery (reduce resistance to 0.5 kg). Take exercise HR at min 2 and 3 of each stage with BP taken at the midpoint of each workload (i.e., begin HR measurement at 1:45, 2:45, 4:45, 5:45, etc. and BP at 2:00, 5:00).

4. The timer should announce the time for the assessment of the respective parameters. Be sure to record the information on the data sheet. Remember to convert the 15 sec HR to beats per minute (bpm).

Discussion Questions

1. What factors can impact the reliability and validity of your HR assessment?
2. The thumb should not be used for HR palpitation. Why?
3. Which HR determination method is closest to a full 60 sec count?
4. What factors can cause changes in resting BP?
5. What information do HR and BP tell us during an exercise test?

Bibliography

ACSM (American College of Sports Medicine). 2010. *ACSM's guidelines for exercise testing and prescription.* 8th ed. Baltimore: Lippincott Williams & Wilkins.

ACSM (American College of Sports Medicine). 2010. *ACSM's resource manual for guidelines for exercise testing and prescription.* 6th ed. Baltimore: Lippincott Williams & Wilkins.

Pina, I.L., G.J. Balady, P. Hanson, A.J. Labovitz, D.W. Madonna, and J. Myers. 1995. Guidelines for exercise testing laboratories. *Circulation* 91: 912-921.

U.S. Department of Health and Human Services. 1996. *Physical activity and health: A report of the Surgeon General.* Washington, DC: International Medical Publishing.

Skinfold and Circumference Assessment Techniques

Purpose

This lab introduces the specific measurement techniques for assessing skinfolds and circumferences.

Materials

- Skinfold calipers
- Gulick tape
- Marker (optional)
- One copy of the Skinfold and Circumference Data Collection Worksheet (appendix B, page 122)

Background Information

As in the previous lab, familiarity with assessment tools and techniques is essential for accurate exercise testing. Through repeated practice with the devices and guidance from a qualified instructor, you can develop the skills necessary to accurately test and measure the specific variables and become proficient in exercise testing.

Body fat levels and fat distribution are recognized as valid predictors of health risks associated with obesity (ACSM 2010). The diseases associated with high levels of body fat include hypertension, coronary artery disease, type 2 diabetes, hyperlipidemia, and certain types of cancers (ACSM 2010, U.S. Department of Health and Human Services 1996).

Skinfold and circumference procedures provide an inexpensive method for identifying obesity risk. **Skinfold calipers** are used to measure the thickness of a double layer of finger-pinched skin and subcutaneous fat. **Gulick tape**, used to measure circumference, is a flexible measuring tape equipped with a spring-loaded attachment at the end that, when pulled out to a specified mark, exerts a fixed amount of tension on the tape. Table 5.1 describes the sites to use for both skinfold and circumference measurements. The ACSM outlines specific procedures for each method (ACSM 2010).

Table 5.1 Standardized Descriptions of Sites for Body Composition Measurements

Skinfold measurement sites	
Abdominal	Measure a perpendicular fold 2 cm to the right of and level with the umbilicus. Be sure that the caliper is not in the umbilicus. Calipers should be applied 1 cm below fingers for each assessment.
Biceps	Measure fold lifted over the belly of the biceps brachii at a level marked 1 cm above the level used for the triceps (see below) and in line with the anterior border of the acromial process and the antecubital fossa.
Triceps	Measure a vertical fold over the belly of the triceps muscle along the posterior midline of the upper arm, half the distance between the acromion and olecranon processes. The arm should be relaxed.
Chest	Measure a diagonal fold along the natural line of the skin one half for men or one third for women the distance between the anterior axillary line and the nipple.
Midaxillary	Measure a vertical fold at the level of the xiphoid process on the midaxillary line.
Subscapular	Measure 2 cm below the inferior angle of the scapula at a 45° angle.
Suprailiac	Measure a diagonal fold in line with the natural angle of the iliac crest along the anterior axillary line immediately above the iliac crest.
Thigh	Measure a vertical fold over the quadriceps muscle on the midline of the thigh, half the distance between the top of the patella and the inguinal crease. The leg should be relaxed.
Medial Calf	Measure a vertical fold lifted at the level of maximum circumference on medial aspect of calf with knee and hip flexed to 90°.
Circumference measurement sites	
Waist	Measure the narrowest part of the torso between the xiphoid process and the umbilicus following exhalation and prior to the next breath.
Hips	Measure the maximal circumference of the buttocks above the gluteal fold. Be sure that the person is standing erect, relaxed, and with feet together.

Procedures

1. In groups of 3 to 5, practice taking skinfolds and circumferences on a partner. Record your own skinfolds and circumferences on the **Skinfolds and Circumference Data Collection Worksheet**.

2. Follow the standard skinfold and circumferential techniques outlined in this lab.

Skinfold Technique

1. Take measurements on the right side of the body.

2. Place the calipers 1 cm away from the thumb and finger, perpendicular to the skinfold and halfway between the crest and base of the fold (figure 5.1).

3. Maintain the pinch while reading the calipers.

4. Wait 1 to 2 seconds (and not longer) before reading the calipers.

5. Take duplicate measures at each site.

6. If measurements do not fall within 2 mm, retest.

7. Rotate through measurement sites or allow time for skin to regain normal texture and thickness.

8. Record the measurements on data sheets.

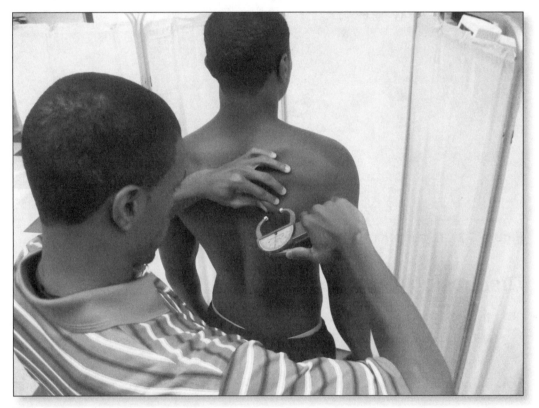

Figure 5.1   Measuring the abdominal site skinfold. Note the placement of calipers with respect to the fingers of the left hand.

Circumference Technique

1. Pull Gulick tape to proper tension (so it is snug) without pinching the skin. Check that the tape is neither indenting the skin nor loose enough to leave gaps between the tape and skin (figure 5.2).

2. Take duplicate measurements at each site.

3. If measurements do not fall within 1 cm, retest.

4. Record the measurements on data sheets.

When assessing body composition using either method, technique accuracy is extremely important. To improve tester accuracy, the ACSM recommends one should train with a skilled technician, routinely practice the techniques, attend workshops, and regularly demonstrate reliability (ACSM 2010).

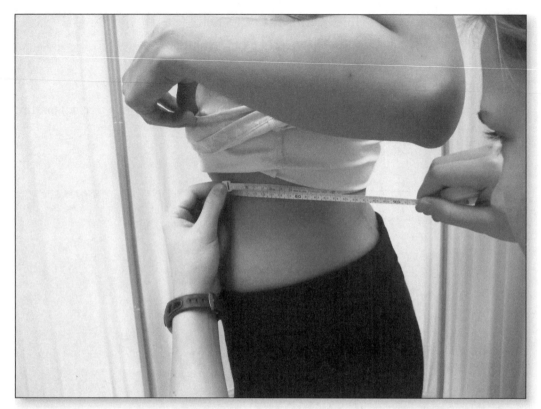

Figure 5.2 Circumference measurement at the waist.

Discussion Questions

1. Describe sources of error when taking skinfolds and circumferences.
2. Why are skinfolds taken on the right side of the body?
3. Why should you wait or rotate through sites when taking measurements?
4. Why should you use a Gulick tape when taking circumference measurements?

References

ACSM (American College of Sports Medicine). 2010. *ACSM's guidelines for exercise testing and prescription.* 8th ed. Baltimore: Lippincott Williams & Wilkins.

U.S. Department of Health and Human Services. 1996. *Physical activity and health: A report of the Surgeon General.* 1st ed. Washington, DC: International Medical Publishing.

Assessing Body Fatness

Purpose

This lab exposes you to field procedures commonly used to assess body fat. You will calculate results from the different equations used to determine body fat.

Materials

- Skinfold calipers
- Gulick tape
- Calculator
- Two copies of the BMI and Body Fatness Data Collection Worksheet (appendix B, page 126)
- Two copies of the Skinfold and Circumference Data Collection Worksheet (appendix B, page 122)

Background Information

We know that a high amount of fat weight (obesity) is a risk factor for heart disease, diabetes, cancer, and other health problems (Howley and Franks 2007). Excess fat weight makes movement inefficient and difficult. A high lean body weight allows the body to accomplish work efficiently and expend more calories even at rest.

The term **body composition** refers to the percentage of body weight that is fat (% body fat) compared with total lean mass. Its measurement is based on the assumption that body weight can be divided into lean body weight and fat weight. Lean body mass encompasses all of the body's nonfat tissues, including the skeleton, water, muscle, connective tissue, organ tissues, and teeth. The fat component includes both the essential and nonessential fat stores. Essential fat includes fat incorporated into organs and tissues; nonessential fat is primarily within adipose tissue. Evaluation of body composition typically is included as part of a health screen or physical fitness assessment.

Body composition can be measured in many ways, including both laboratory and field techniques. Although they are not as accurate, anthropometric methods provide a more practical and less expensive alternative than hydrostatic weighing to estimate body composition. Thus, this lab will focus on formulas and equations involving skinfolds, circumference, waist-to-hip ratio, and body mass index (BMI).

Interpreting Body Composition Data

It is important to distinguish between being *overweight* and being *overfat* (obese). Overweight is defined as exceeding the normal or standard weight for a specific height and skeletal frame size, when grouped by gender. Being overweight is not necessarily undesirable, especially when the lean body mass is high. Measuring body density and calculating fat weight and lean body weight allow a more accurate method of estimating desired weight rather than using height-and-weight tables, which do not determine fat and lean weight. Overfat, or obesity, is defined as the state of having excess body fat. Although no universal agreement exists on the specific percentage of body fat that constitutes obesity, it is recommended that men and women maintain body fat percentages of 10 to 22% and 20 to 32%, respectively.

Interpretation of body composition must be individualized to each person. As a fitness professional you should be aware of the wide range of normal values and should not encourage all participants to achieve the same particular value. The principle of variability is important. Humans vary widely on any trait that can be measured and body composition is no exception. You must recognize this and take it into account in interpreting body composition data.

Anthropometric Definitions

- **Body mass index.** The body mass index (BMI), or Quetelet index, examines body weight relative to height. It is calculated by dividing body weight (in kg) by height (in m) squared (wt/ht^2). BMI is a good indicator of total body composition in population-based studies and is related to health outcomes. As the BMI increases, mortality from heart disease, cancer, and diabetes also increases. Significant increases in risk begin at a BMI of about 30.0 kg/m^2 for men and women.

- **Circumference.** Measurement of body girths may be reasonably accurate in estimating body fat (from prediction equations) in unfit subjects. These measurements, however, do not detect changes in body composition over time when lean tissue increases and fat mass decreases. Thus, for consistent evaluation of body fat percentage, they appear to be impractical.

- **Waist-to-hip ratio.** As mentioned earlier, excessive body fat is a health hazard. The distribution of body fat also affects a person's health. Levels of subcutaneous body fat levels in the upper body (waist measurement) and lower body (hip measurement) are distributed differently by sex, age, body type, and activity level. Fat in the abdomen (upper body) is associated with greater morbidity and mortality than is fat distributed below the abdomen (lower body). Ideally, waist circumference should be smaller than hip circumference. Waist-to-hip ratios above .95 for men and .85 for women are considered to place the person at significantly increased risk for obesity-related health problems.

- **Skinfold.** Results from the skinfold method of estimating body composition correlate fairly well with hydrostatic weighing. Measuring the thickness of skinfolds involves grasping a fold of skin and fat and holding it away from the underlying muscle. The reliability of skinfold measurements depends on meticulous attention to detail in the techniques. Practice the techniques extensively and be precise in measuring the exact anatomical locations indicated.

You can use skinfold measurement values in several ways: You can total the values from several sites to arrive at the sum of skinfolds. You can use the sum of skinfolds to rate individuals within a given group. You can also use the sum of skinfolds to evaluate changes in body fat following dietary restriction, exercise conditioning programs, or a combination of them. You can also use skinfold measurements with mathematical equations to predict percentage of body fat. Keep in mind that equations derived from one segment of the population do a poor job of predicting percent fat for other populations; the equations are applicable only to groups similar in age and activity level to those from which the equations are derived. When well-trained, experienced technicians perform the measurements, skinfold-based estimates of body fat percentages are generally within 3.5% of measurements obtained using the underwater weighing technique.

Procedures

1. Follow the appropriate skinfold procedures (page 36) and circumferential technique (page 37) found in lab 5.
2. Record the participant's weight, age, skinfold measurements, and circumferences on the **Skinfold and Circumference Data Collection Worksheet**. Do this for one male and one female.
3. Complete the BMI Calculation and Risk Classification sections on the **BMI and Body Fatness Data Collection Worksheet**.
4. Determine the BMI classification according to table 6.1.
5. Use appropriate anthropometric equations (male or female) from appendix E (page 146) to calculate body density. Use the 7-site and both 3-site formulas.
6. Once you have calculated body density use the Brozek or Siri body density conversion formula to calculate the percentage of body fat (see appendix E, page 146).
7. Determine each subject's body fat percentile and rating according to table 6.2.
8. Determine each subject's fat mass and lean mass from each equation. (Multiply % fat by total body weight for fat mass weight; total body weight minus fat weight equals lean mass weight.)

Discussion Questions

1. What are the similarities and differences between the various anthropometric measures discussed in this lab?
2. Which of the body composition assessment equations discussed in this lab are most valid or reliable? Are some equations better or worse for specific age groups and populations? If yes, for what age groups and populations are these equations most appropriate?
3. What professional considerations are appropriate when using these measures in a field setting?

Table 6.1 Body Mass Index, Waist Circumference Disease Risk[†] Classification, and Predicted Body Fat Percentage

BMI (men)	Classification	Risk level by waist circumference		Predicted body fat percentage by age[‡]		
		≤102 cm	≥102 cm	20-39 yr	40-59 yr	60-79 yr
<18.5	Underweight	...	...	<8%	<11%	<13%
18.5-24.9	Normal[§]	...	...	8-19%	11-21%	13-24%
25.0-29.9	Overweight	Increased	High	20-24%	22-27%	25-29%
30.0-34.9	Class 1 obesity	High	Very high	≥25%	≥28%	≥30%
35.0-39.9	Class 2 obesity	Very high	Very high			
≥40.0	Class 3 obesity	Extremely high	Extremely high			
BMI (women)	**Classification**	**≤88 cm**	**≥88 cm**	**20-39 yr**	**40-59 yr**	**60-79 yr**
<18.5	Underweight	...	...	<21%	<23%	<24%
18.5-24.9	Normal[§]	...	...	21-32%	23-33%	24-35%
25.0-29.9	Overweight	Increased	High	33-38%	34-39%	36-41%
30.0-34.9	Class 1 obesity	High	Very high	≥39%	≥40%	≥42%
35.0-39.9	Class 2 obesity	Very high	Very high			
≥40.0	Class 3 obesity	Extremely high	Extremely high			

A gender-neutral value for waist circumference (>100 cm) has also been suggested as an index of obesity.

[†]Disease risk for type 2 diabetes, hypertension, and cardiovascular disease. Ellipses indicate no additional risk at these levels of BMI was assigned.

[§]Increased waist circumference can also be a marker for increased risk even in persons of normal weight.

[‡]Standard error of estimate is ±5% for predicting percent body fat from BMI (based on a four-compartment estimate of body fat percentage).

Adapted, by permission, from American College of Sports Medicine, 2010, *ACSM's guidelines for exercise testing and prescription,* 8th ed. (Baltimore: Lippincott, Williams & Wilkins), 63, 64.

4. In procedure 4, you calculated body composition using the same data using different equations (7 site vs. 3 site). Compare the results from each equation. Do the results differ? If yes, why?

Bibliography

ACSM (American College of Sports Medicine). 2010. *ACSM's guidelines for exercise testing and prescription.* 8th ed. Baltimore: Lippincott Williams & Wilkins.

ACSM (American College of Sports Medicine). 2010. *Resource manual for guidelines for exercise testing and prescription.* 6th ed. Baltimore: Lippincott Williams & Wilkins.

Howley, E.T., and B.D. Franks. 2007. *Fitness professional's handbook.* 5th ed. Champaign, IL: Human Kinetics.

Table 6.2 Body Composition Chart (Values Expressed in % Body Fat)

Percentile	Rating	Age (yr)					
		20-29	30-39	40-49	50-59	60-69	70-79
Men							
99	Very lean	4.2	7.0	9.2	10.9	11.5	13.6
95		6.3	9.9	12.8	14.4	15.5	15.2
90		7.9	11.9	14.9	16.7	17.6	17.8
85		9.2	13.3	16.3	18.0	18.8	19.2
80	Excellent	10.5	14.5	17.4	19.1	19.7	20.4
75		11.5	15.5	18.4	19.9	20.6	21.1
70		12.7	16.5	19.1	20.7	21.3	21.6
65		13.9	17.4	19.9	21.3	22.0	22.5
60	Good	14.8	18.2	20.6	22.1	22.6	23.1
55		15.8	19.0	21.3	22.7	23.2	23.7
50		16.6	19.7	21.9	23.2	23.7	24.1
45		17.4	20.4	22.6	23.9	24.4	24.4
40	Fair	18.6	21.3	23.4	24.6	25.2	24.8
35		19.6	22.1	24.1	25.3	26.0	25.4
30		20.6	23.0	24.8	26.0	26.7	26.0
25		21.9	23.9	25.7	26.8	27.5	26.7
20	Poor	23.1	24.9	26.6	27.8	28.4	27.6
15		24.6	26.2	27.7	28.9	29.4	28.9
10		26.3	27.8	29.2	30.3	30.9	30.4
5		28.9	30.2	31.2	32.5	32.9	32.4
1	Very poor	33.3	34.3	35.0	36.4	36.8	35.5
Women							
99	Very lean	9.8	11.0	12.6	14.6	13.9	14.6
95		13.6	14.0	15.6	17.2	17.7	16.6
90		14.8	15.6	17.2	19.4	19.8	20.3
85		15.8	16.6	18.6	20.9	21.4	23.0
80	Excellent	16.5	17.4	19.8	22.5	23.2	24.0
75		17.3	18.2	20.8	23.8	24.8	25.0
70		18.0	19.1	21.9	25.1	25.9	26.2
65		18.7	20.0	22.8	26.0	27.0	27.7
60	Good	19.4	20.8	23.8	27.0	27.9	28.6
55		20.1	21.7	24.8	27.9	28.7	29.7
50		21.0	22.6	25.6	28.8	29.8	30.4
45		21.9	23.5	26.5	29.7	30.6	31.3
40	Fair	22.7	24.6	27.6	30.4	31.3	31.8
35		23.6	25.6	28.5	31.4	32.5	32.7
30		24.5	26.7	29.6	32.5	33.3	33.9
25		25.9	27.7	30.7	33.4	34.3	35.3
20	Poor	27.1	29.1	31.9	34.5	35.4	36.0
15		28.9	30.9	33.5	35.6	36.2	37.4
10		31.4	33.0	35.4	36.7	37.3	38.2
5		35.2	35.8	37.4	38.3	39.0	39.3
1	Very poor	38.9	39.4	39.8	40.4	40.8	40.5

Reprinted with permission from the Cooper Institute, Dallas, Texas. For more information: www.cooperinstitute.org.

Submaximal Exercise Test Protocols

Purpose

This lab presents two types of submaximal exercise test protocols for determining cardiovascular fitness levels (the Åstrand-Ryhming test and the YMCA Submaximal Cycle Ergometer Protocol) and emphasizes practice of these protocols.

Materials

- Cycle ergometer or treadmill
- Sphygmomanometer
- Stethoscope
- Stopwatch
- RPE scale
- One copy of the Åstrand-Ryhming Data Collection Worksheet (appendix B, page 124)
- Copy of the YMCA Test Data Collection Worksheet (appendix B, page 125)
- ECG (if available)

Background Information

Exercise scientists generally consider the best indicator of cardiovascular fitness to be the body's ability to take in and utilize oxygen. The measurement of this ability is known as **maximal oxygen consumption**, or $\dot{V}O_2$**max.** The most widely accepted predictor of cardiovascular fitness is one's HR response to submaximal work. Tables 7.1 and 7.2 present predicted $\dot{V}O_2$max values based on HR responses to specific workloads on a cycle ergometer in men and women, respectively.

Once again, because numerous pharmacological agents can affect HR, it is important to identify the medications that a participant is taking and determine whether or not medication is impacting HR and or BP. Appendix C contains a list of pharmacological agents and their effects on cardiorespiratory responses to exercise. For participants who are taking medications that alter HR responses, it is unreliable to use submaximal HR as a predictor of $\dot{V}O_2$max.

Table 7.1 Prediction of Maximal Oxygen Uptake in Men From HR and Workload on a Cycle Ergometer

HR	300 kpm/min	600 kpm/min	900 kpm/min	1,200 kpm/min	1,500 kpm/min	HR	300 kpm/min	600 kpm/min	900 kpm/min	1,200 kpm/min	1,500 kpm/min
120	2.2	3.5	4.8			148		2.4	3.2	4.3	5.4
121	2.2	3.4	4.7			149		2.3	3.2	4.3	5.4
122	2.2	3.4	4.6			150		2.3	3.2	4.2	5.3
123	2.1	3.4	4.6			151		2.3	3.1	4.2	5.2
124	2.1	3.3	4.5	6.0		152		2.3	3.1	4.1	5.2
125	2.0	3.2	4.4	5.9		153		2.2	3.0	4.1	5.1
126	2.0	3.2	4.4	5.8		154		2.2	3.0	4.0	5.1
127	2.0	3.1	4.3	5.7		155		2.2	3.0	4.0	5.0
128	2.0	3.1	4.2	5.6		156		2.2	2.9	4.0	5.0
129	1.9	3.0	4.2	5.6		157		2.1	2.9	3.9	4.9
130	1.9	3.0	4.1	5.5		158		2.1	2.9	3.9	4.9
131	1.9	2.9	4.0	5.4		159		2.1	2.8	3.8	4.8
132	1.8	2.9	4.0	5.3		160		2.1	2.8	3.8	4.8
133	1.8	2.8	3.9	5.3		161		2.0	2.8	3.7	4.7
134	1.8	2.8	3.9	5.2		162		2.0	2.8	3.7	4.6
135	1.7	2.8	3.8	5.1		163		2.0	2.8	3.7	4.6
136	1.7	2.7	3.8	5.0		164		2.0	2.7	3.6	4.5
137	1.7	2.7	3.7	5.0		165		2.0	2.7	3.6	4.5
138	1.6	2.7	3.7	4.9		166		1.9	2.7	3.6	4.5
139	1.6	2.6	3.6	4.8		167		1.9	2.6	3.5	4.4
140	1.6	2.6	3.6	4.8	6.0	168		1.9	2.6	3.5	4.4
141		2.6	3.5	4.7	5.9	169		1.9	2.6	3.5	4.3
142		2.5	3.5	4.6	5.8	170		1.8	2.6	3.4	4.3
143		2.5	3.4	4.6	5.7						
144		2.5	3.4	4.5	5.7						
145		2.4	3.4	4.5	5.6						
146		2.4	3.3	4.4	5.6						
147		2.4	3.3	4.4	5.5						

The value should be corrected for age using the factor given in table 7.3.

Adapted, by permission, from P.O. Åstrand, 1960, "Aerobic work capacity in men and women with special references to age," *Acta Physiologica Scandanavia* 49 (suppl 169): 45-60.

Maximal oxygen consumption may be defined as the maximal rate at which the body can take up, distribute, and use oxygen in the performance of large-muscle-mass exercise. For muscular work lasting more than 6 min at rates for which anaerobic sources of energy are not exceeded, there exists a highest level of work at which the body reaches its maximum capacity to supply oxygen. Levels of $\dot{V}O_2$max are observed after the participant's workload is increased progressively until it exceeds the capacity of the oxygen uptake and requires anaerobic sources of power in the final spurt. When oxygen uptake can no longer increase despite the fact that work can continue

Table 7.2 Prediction of Maximal Oxygen Uptake in Women From HR and Workload on a Cycle Ergometer

HR	300 kpm/ min	450 kpm/ min	600 kpm/ min	750 kpm/ min	900 kpm/ min	HR	300 kpm/ min	450 kpm/ min	600 kpm/ min	750 kpm/ min	900 kpm/ min
120	2.6	3.4	4.1	4.8		146	1.6	2.2	2.6	3.2	3.7
121	2.5	3.3	4.0	4.8		147	1.6	2.1	2.6	3.1	3.6
122	2.5	3.2	3.9	4.7		148	1.6	2.1	2.6	3.1	3.6
123	2.4	3.1	3.9	4.6		149		2.1	2.6	3.0	3.5
124	2.4	3.1	3.8	4.5		150		2.0	2.5	3.0	3.5
125	2.3	3.0	3.7	4.4		151		2.0	2.5	3.0	3.4
126	2.3	3.0	3.6	4.3		152		2.0	2.5	2.9	3.4
127	2.2	2.9	3.5	4.2		153		2.0	2.4	2.9	3.3
128	2.2	2.8	3.5	4.2	4.8	154		2.0	2.4	2.8	3.3
129	2.2	2.8	3.4	4.1	4.8	155		1.9	2.4	2.8	3.2
130	2.1	2.7	3.4	4.0	4.7	156		1.9	2.3	2.8	3.2
131	2.1	2.7	3.4	4.0	4.6	157		1.9	2.3	2.7	3.2
132	2.0	2.7	3.3	3.9	4.5	158		1.8	2.3	2.7	3.1
133	2.0	2.6	3.2	3.8	4.4	159		1.8	2.2	2.7	3.1
134	2.0	2.6	3.2	3.8	4.4	160		1.8	2.2	2.6	3.0
135	2.0	2.6	3.1	3.7	4.3	161		1.8	2.2	2.6	3.0
136	1.9	2.5	3.1	3.6	4.2	162		1.8	2.2	2.6	3.0
137	1.9	2.5	3.0	3.6	4.2	163		1.7	2.2	2.6	2.9
138	1.8	2.4	3.0	3.5	4.1	164		1.7	2.1	2.5	2.9
139	1.8	2.4	2.9	3.5	4.0	165		1.7	2.1	2.5	2.9
140	1.8	2.4	2.8	3.4	4.0	166		1.7	2.1	2.5	2.8
141	1.8	2.3	2.8	3.4	3.9	167		1.6	2.1	2.4	2.8
142	1.7	2.3	2.8	3.3	3.9	168		1.6	2.0	2.4	2.8
143	1.7	2.2	2.7	3.3	3.8	169		1.6	2.0	2.4	2.8
144	1.7	2.2	2.7	3.2	3.8	170		1.6	2.0	2.4	2.7
145	1.6	2.2	2.7	3.2	3.7						

The value should be corrected for age using the factor given in table 7.3.

Adapted, by permission, from P.O. Åstrand, 1960, "Aerobic work capacity in men and women with special references to age," *Acta Physiologica Scandanavia* 49 (suppl 169): 45-60.

at higher levels for a short time because of anaerobic power sources, the participant has reached a plateau for maximal oxygen uptake (aerobic capacity). Every person has a measurable upper limit of oxygen uptake, which correlates with his or her ability to do aerobic work.

Factors Affecting $\dot{V}O_2$max

A person's $\dot{V}O_2$max level depends on body build and composition and is affected by the following factors:

1. **Sex.** Comparatively, the typical female will have a lower $\dot{V}O_2$max than the typical male.

2. **Age.** Maximal oxygen uptake ($\dot{V}O_2$max) decreases by 10% per decade in men and women regardless of age and exercise activity (Hawkins & Wiswell, 2003).

3. **Size.** A person's maximal oxygen uptake is directly proportional to height and body surface area.

4. **Weight.** Maximal oxygen uptake is proportional to a person's weight.

5. **Lean body mass.** $\dot{V}O_2$max correlates 0.63 with body mass, 0.85 with fat-free body mass, and 0.91 with active muscle tissue.

6. **Bed rest.** Enforced bed rest of 3 weeks reduces maximal oxygen uptake by approximately 17%.

7. **Altitude.** At an altitude of 4,000 m $\dot{V}O_2$max is reduced by approximately 26%. The reduction increases as altitude increases.

8. **Geography.** $\dot{V}O_2$max is reduced for residents of temperate or tropical areas as compared with those living in circumpolar regions.

Maximal oxygen uptake is not affected by the following:

1. Ingestion of a small meal (up to about 750 kcal)

2. Exposure to heat stress up to 90 °F

3. Whether the participant warms up before exercise (duration of warm-up exercise can vary)

4. Speed of exercise (rate of work can be slow, moderate, or fast)

5. Repetition (retests at intervals of 20-30 min show similar results)

Maximal oxygen uptake can increase with physical conditioning or decrease with inactivity. The limiting factors may be one or both of the following:

1. The capacity of the respiratory and circulatory systems to take up and transport oxygen, a process that is dependent on alveolar ventilation, diffusing capacity of the lungs, and capacity of the blood flow for transporting oxygen from the lungs to the capillaries

2. The capacity of the working muscles to receive and use oxygen

For participants older than 30 yr, table 7.3 presents the correction factors for the predicted $\dot{V}O_2$max values found in tables 7.1 and 7.2. To correct for a specific age, multiply the corresponding correction factor by the value obtained from table 7.1 or 7.2. This corrected $\dot{V}O_2$max value can then be used to determine the fitness classification of the participant. Table 7.4 presents the $\dot{V}O_2$max fitness classifications by sex and age group.

Measuring $\dot{V}O_2$max

A maximal oxygen consumption test requires that the participant exert maximal effort in performing physical work, generally on a treadmill or bike, to exhaustion. The test begins with a relatively light workload and progresses, with increases every 2 to 3 min, to a workload that the participant can no longer sustain. This requires great

Table 7.3 Correction Factors for Predicted Maximal Oxygen Uptake

Age	Factor	HRmax	Factor
15	1.10	210	1.12
25	1.00	200	1.00
35	0.87	190	0.93
40	0.83	180	0.83
45	0.78	170	0.75
50	0.75	160	0.69
55	0.71	150	0.64
60	0.68		
65	0.65		

Factor to be used for correction of predicted maximal oxygen uptake (a) when the participant is older than 30 to 35 yr of age, or (b) when the participant's HRmax is known. Multiply the actual factor by the value obtained from table 7.1 or table 7.2.

Adapted, by permission, from P.O. Åstrand, 1960, "Aerobic work capacity in men and women with special references to age," *Acta Physiologica Scandanavia* 49 (suppl 169): 45-60.

Table 7.4 Classification of Maximal Oxygen Uptake (Maximal Aerobic Power) by Age Group

Age	Low	Somewhat low	Average	High	Very high
Women					
20-29	≤1.69 ≤28	1.70-1.99 29-34	2.00-2.49 35-43	2.50-2.79 44-48	≥2.80 ≥49
30-39	≤1.59 ≤27	1.60-1.89 28-33	1.90-2.39 34-41	2.40-2.69 42-47	≥2.70 ≥48
40-49	≤1.49 ≤25	1.50-1.79 26-31	1.80-2.29 32-40	2.30-2.59 41-45	≥2.60 ≥46
50-65	≤1.29 ≤21	1.30-1.59 22-28	1.60-2.09 29-36	2.10-2.39 37-41	≥2.40 ≥42
Men					
20-29	≤2.79 ≤38	2.80-3.09 39-43	3.10-3.69 48-51	3.70-3.99 52-56	≥4.00 ≥57
30-39	≤2.49 ≤34	2.50-2.79 35-39	2.80-3.39 40-47	3.40-3.69 48-51	≥3.70 ≥52
40-49	≤2.19 ≤30	2.20-2.49 31-35	2.50-3.09 36-43	3.10-3.39 44-47	≥3.40 ≥48
50-59	≤1.89 ≤25	1.90-2.19 26-31	2.20-2.79 32-39	2.80-3.09 40-43	≥3.10 ≥44
60-69	≤1.59 ≤21	1.60-1.89 22-26	1.90-2.49 27-35	2.50-2.79 36-39	≥2.80 ≥40

The upper number, e.g., 1.69, refers to maximal oxygen uptake in L/min. The lower number, e.g., 28, refers to ml/kg · min. Weights used were 58 kg for females and 72 kg for males.

Adapted, by permission, from P.O. Åstrand, 1960, "Aerobic work capacity in men and women with special references to age," *Acta Physiologica Scandanavia* 49 (suppl 169): 45-60.

effort by the participant. To ensure accuracy, the tester evaluates criteria to ensure that the participant has achieved a maximal level of oxygen consumption. The four most relevant criteria are

1. the plateau of oxygen consumption,
2. the attainment of respiratory exchange ratios of 1:1 or higher,
3. the attainment of age-predicted HR, and
4. the exhaustion of the participant.

Spirometry

Maximal oxygen uptake can be measured by **open-circuit spirometry** (a method of indirect calorimetry in which the subject breathes air from the atmosphere) or can be predicted from the peak exercise time or power output achieved during a standard maximal exercise test protocol (i.e., Bruce protocol). It can also be predicted from submaximal exercise tests.

The open-circuit spirometry method of measuring oxygen consumption is the most accurate means currently available for determining a person's aerobic capacity during exercise. The participant inhales ambient air composed of 20.93% oxygen, 0.03-0.04% carbon dioxide, and 79.04% nitrogen during exercise. Because the body uses the oxygen, the exhaled gases will contain less oxygen and more carbon dioxide than the inhaled air. The equipment for open-circuit spirometry is expensive and specialized and is not generally available to health and fitness specialists; therefore it will not be discussed further in this lab.

Submaximal Exercise Tests

A $\dot{V}O_2$ max test is not practical for a large population, nor is it always safe for all participants. With this in mind, exercise technicians have developed a submaximal test that should accurately estimate a person's maximal $\dot{V}O_2$. These submaximal tests use HR responses to incremental workloads to predict percentages of $\dot{V}O_2$ max. As workload increases, HR increases proportionately (positive linear relationship). Once you have established a participant's HR responses to a series of submaximal loads, you can use the slope of the line created by the HR responses to those workloads and extrapolate to the participant's age-predicted maximal HR to a prediction of $\dot{V}O_2$ max. This prediction is an estimate of $\dot{V}O_2$ max. The underlying basis of submaximal tests involving HR, $\dot{V}O_2$, and workload are shown in figure 7.1.

The Åstrand-Ryhming test and the YMCA Submaximal Cycle Ergometer Protocol are procedures that fitness professionals commonly use to predict $\dot{V}O_2$ max.

Rating of Perceived Exertion

Another means of determining whether a participant has reached maximal oxygen uptake is through the use of a scale known as the rating of perceived exertion (RPE). This scale serves as a subjective measure of the participant's sense of effort. Someone who is performing maximal work will report maximal effort; thus this scale provides further support for the accuracy of a maximal effort test. In addition, fitness professionals can use RPE to prescribe exercise intensity.

Because maximal HR varies greatly among participants during exercise, it is helpful to be able to evaluate RPE to assess whether a test is truly maximal and when a participant is approaching maximum exercise. RPE from the category scale correlates

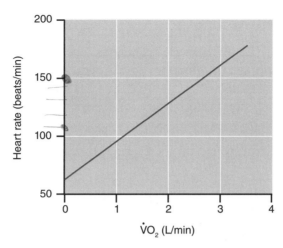

Figure 7.1   The linear relationship between HR and workload increases. When you measure HR at each stage of a submaximal exercise test, you can predict a person's $\dot{V}O_2$ max by extrapolating the maximal workload to the age-predicted maximal HR.

Reprinted, by permission, from F. Cerny and H. Burton, 2001, *Exercise physiology for health care professionals* (Champaign, IL: Human Kinetics), 302.

closely with several exercise variables, including percentage of $\dot{V}O_2$**peak** ($\dot{V}O_2$peak is used to refer to the highest $\dot{V}O_2$ achieved during a max test. Often this term describes $\dot{V}O_2$ when the criterion for $\dot{V}O_2$max is not met), percentage of heart rate reserve (HRR), minute ventilation, and blood lactate levels.

During most exercise testing, the RPE scale is an accurate gauge of impeding fatigue. Clinical experience indicates, however, that 5 to 10% of test participants unfamiliar with the scale tend to underestimate or suppress RPE below expected levels during the early and middle stages of testing. For this reason, it is important that the participant you are testing has a clear understanding of the RPE scale and how to gauge effort. To communicate this thoroughly, first make sure that you understand the RPE scale. Then, before beginning the test, state the following to the subject:

> *"While you are participating in exercise, it is quite common to have a sense of how hard you are working. I would like you to consider the total amount of exertion you feel, taking into account all sensations of physical stress, effort, and fatigue in your whole body."*

Procedures

1. Determine the estimated relative and absolute $\dot{V}O_2$max from each test.

2. Before beginning the procedures, review general indications for stopping an exercise test in low-risk adults and absolute and relative indications for terminating exercise testing on pages 83 and 119 of *ACSM's Guidelines for Exercise Testing and Prescription, Eighth Edition.*

Following are the steps in administering two different submaximal cycle ergometer tests.

Åstrand-Ryhming Test

1. Adjust the seat height on the cycle **ergometer.** The participant should sit upright and when the foot is at the bottom of the pedaling stroke, that leg should be slightly bent at the knee, 5°.

2. Record the participant's weight, age, resting HR, and resting BP on the **Åstrand-Ryhming Test Data Collection Worksheet.**

3. Have the participant warm up for 2 to 3 min by pedaling at 50 rpm with no resistance.

4. Instruct the participant to continue pedaling, and immediately set the resistance according to the following scale.

   Unconditioned participant

   Male 300 kgm/min (1 kp = 50 Watts) or 600 kgm/min (2 kp = 100 Watts)

   Female 300 kgm/min (1 kp = 50 Watts) or 450 kgm/min (1.5 kp = 75 Watts)

   Conditioned participant

   Male 600 kgm/min (2 kp = 100 Watts) or 900 kgm/min (3 kp = 150 Watts)

   Female 450 kgm/min (1.5 kp = 75 Watts) or 600 kgm/min (2 kp = 100 Watts)

5. Monitor HR, BP, and RPE during the 6 min of exercise. On the worksheet, record the HR during the last 15 sec of each min (i.e., 1:45, 2.45); record the BP during the last 30 sec of each 2 min phase (i.e., 1:30, 3:30); record RPE during the last 15 sec of the phase.

6. The timer should announce the time for the assessment of the respective parameters. Be sure to record the information on the data sheet. Remember to convert the 15 sec HR to beats per minute (bpm).

7. Continue by performing one of the following steps:

   a. After the 6 min testing period, if the participant *has* reached an average target HR of between 125 and 170 bpm, begin a 4 min cool-down stage with 0 resistance. Record HR, BP, and RPE after each minute. Talk with the participant about any problems that may have occurred.

   b. After the 6 min testing period, if the participant *has not* reached an average target HR of between 125 and 170 bpm, continue the test for an additional 1 min, increasing the workload by 0.5 kp until the participant attains an HR of at least 125 bpm. Increase the resistance by 0.5 kp each 1 min until the participant attains an HR of at least 125 bpm. At the end of each I min, take and record HR and BP. Once the participant *has* reached an average target HR of between 125 and 170 bpm, begin a 4 min cool-down stage with 0 resistance. Record HR, BP, and RPE after each 1 min. Talk with the participant about any problems that may have occurred.

8. Refer to table 7.1 or 7.2 to obtain the maximal oxygen uptake (L/min) for the participant based on the average of the HRs in min 5 and 6 (or, if step 7b were taken, average from the last 2 min).

9. Correct the value obtained from table 7.1 or 7.2 for age using the factor given in table 7.3.

10. After obtaining the absolute maximal oxygen uptake, determine the relative maximal oxygen uptake.

11. Refer to table 7.4 to determine the subject's fitness level.

YMCA Test

A portion of the following instructions for the YMCA test has been adapted with permission from B.D. Franks and E.T. Howley, 1989, *Fitness leader's handbook* (Champaign, IL: Human Kinetics), 87.

1. Record the participant's weight, age, resting HR, and resting BP on the **YMCA Test Data Collection Worksheet.**

2. Complete the calculations for age-predicted maximum HR (HRmax) and target HR.

   a. Estimate the participant's HRmax (220 – age = bpm).

   b. Determine 85% of the participant's HRmax (HRmax $\times$ .85 = 85% HRmax) or 70% of HR reserve [(HRmax – resting HR) $\times$ (.70 + resting HR)].

3. Review the procedure with the participant:

   "This is a two- to four-stage test, with each stage lasting 3 minutes. I will measure your heart rate during the last 15 to 30 seconds of minutes 2 and 3 of each stage, and I will measure your blood pressure and rating of perceived exertion during the last minute of each stage. If the two heart rate measurements I take in each stage are not within 6 beats per minute of each other, I will add time to the stage in 1-minute increments until your heart rate reaches a steady rate."

4. Set and record the seat height (the participant should sit upright, and when the foot is at the bottom of the pedaling stroke, that leg should be slightly bent at the knee, about 5°).

5. Start the metronome. Set it at 100 bpm so that one foot is at the bottom of the pedaling stroke on each beat, resulting in 50 complete rrpm.

6. Have the participant begin pedaling, with no resistance, in rhythm with the metronome. Continue this pace for 2 to 3 min for the participant to warm up.

7. As soon as the participant has maintained the warm-up pace for 2 to 3 min, set the resistance according to the YMCA cycle protocol. Check the resistance setting (it may drift) and observe the participant for signs or symptoms that require termination of the test. *[handwritten: warm up 2-3 minute]*

8. Monitor HR, BP, and RPE during the 6 min of exercise. On the worksheet, record the HR during the last 15 sec of the second and third min of each stage min (i.e., 1:45, 2.45, 4:45, 5:45, etc.); record the BP during the last 30 sec of each 3 min phase (i.e., 2:30, 5:30, etc); record RPE during the last 15 sec of each stage. *[handwritten: 1:45 2:45 of each stage record]*

9. The timer should announce the time for the assessment of the respective parameters. Be sure to record the information on the **YMCA Test Data Collection Worksheet**. Remember to convert the 15 sec HR to beats per minute (bpm).

10. Continue until the participant reaches target HR by performing one of the following steps:

    a. If the two HRs obtained in the stage *are* within 6 bpm of each other (referred to as steady-state), increase the workload for the next stage according to the steady-state HR attained. See YMCA Protocol (table 7.5).

    b. If the HRs *are not* within 6 bpm of each other, continue the stage, measuring HR at the end of the additional minute until the participant achieves steady state, then increase the workload to the next stage according to the steady-state HR attained. See YMCA Protocol (table 7.5).

11. Once the target HR is reached, end the testing stage and begin the cool-down by performing one of the following substeps:

    a. Have the participant continue pedaling and reduce the resistance to a work rate equal to or less than that used in the first stage. Continue monitoring for at least 4 min of active recovery, taking HR and BP each 1 min.

    b. If the participant is experiencing signs of discomfort or emergency symptoms, perform a passive cool-down (have the participant cease physical activity), monitoring the participant for at least 4 min and taking HR and BP each 1 min.

12. Plot the HRs (Y-axis) obtained against the work rates (X-axis) from the last minute of each stage on a graph. Draw a horizontal line across the chart for the age-predicted maximum heart rate. Then draw a line of best fit through

Table 7.5 YMCA Protocol

Set the first work rate at 150 kgm/min (0.5 kg at 50 rpm).		
If the HR in the third minute of the first stage is	then set the work rate for the next stage at	
	Stage	Work rate
<80	second stage at	750 kgm/min (2.5 kg at 50 rpm)
	third stage (if required)	900 kgm/min (3.0 kg)
	fourth stage (if required)	1,050 kgm/min (3.5 kg)
80-89	second stage	600 kgm/min (2.0 kg at 50 rpm)
	third stage (if required)	750 kgm/min (3.0 kg)
	fourth stage (if required)	900 kgm/min (3.5 kg)
90-100	second stage	450 kgm/min (1.5 kg at 50 rpm)
	third stage (if required)	600 kgm/min (3.0 kg)
	fourth stage (if required)	750 kgm/min (3.5 kg)
>100	second stage	300 kgm/min (1.0 kg at 50 rpm)
	third stage (if required)	450 kgm/min (3.0 kg)
	fourth stage (if required)	600 kgm/min (3.5 kg)

*Note: kgm is also referred to as kpm.

Based on L.A. Golding 2000.

the HR points up to the age-predicted HRmax. Draw a line straight down from this intersection to estimate the work rate that would have been attained had the participant achieved HRmax. The value displayed is the estimated maximal work rate the participant would have achieved during a maximal stress test.

Arm Exercise Test Protocol

The arm exercise test is designed for people who are nonambulatory or those who perform dynamic upper-body work during occupational or recreational activities and are interested in assessing upper-body fitness. Be sure to gather the demographic and resting data described earlier (the date; the participant's name, age, resting HR, resting BP, age-predicted HRmax, and target HR) before testing.

When using an arm exercise protocol,

1. begin with no resistance on the flywheel; then increase 25 Watts (150 kgm/min) every 2 min continuous stage without stopping (BP can be difficult to obtain), or

2. begin with no resistance on the flywheel; then increase 25 Watts (150 kgm/min) every 2 min discontinuous stage (better tolerated by participants and allows for more frequent, more reliable BP measures).

When assessing cardiorespiratory fitness with arm ergometry, remember the following factors:

- BP drops rapidly immediately after termination of upright arm-cranking exercise. Thus, an accurate measure of BP must be taken immediately.
- Maximal arm exercise $\dot{V}O_2$ is usually 70 to 80% of that determined from leg exercise.
- Values of HRmax are similar to or slightly lower than those achieved during treadmill or cycle ergometer exercise.

Discussion Questions

1. What is the purpose of determining cardiorespiratory fitness?
2. What is the most reliable and valid measure of cardiorespiratory fitness?
3. Why is it acceptable to use HR as a predictor of cardiorespiratory fitness?
4. What is the fitness classification of the participant being tested? (See table 6.1 for men and table 6.2 for women.)
5. What factors may affect the results of these predictions?
6. What are the determinants of oxygen uptake?
7. What are the objective criteria for terminating a maximal oxygen consumption test?

Bibliography

ACSM (American College of Sports Medicine). 2010. *ACSM's Guidelines for Exercise Testing and Prescription.* 8th ed. Baltimore: Lippincott Williams & Wilkins.

Borg, G. 1998. *Borg's perceived exertion and pain scales.* Champaign, IL: Human Kinetics.

Bruce, R.A., F. Kusumi, and D. Hosmer. 1973. Maximal oxygen intake and nomographic assessment of functional aerobic impairment in cardiovascular disease. *American Heart Journal* 85: 545-62.

Golding, L. 2000. *YMCA fitness testing and assessment manual.* 4th ed. Champaign, IL: Human Kinetics.

Hawkins, S.A., and R.A. Wiswell. 2003. Rate and mechanism of maximal oxygen consumption decline with aging. *Sports Medicine* 33: 877-88.

Howley, E.T. and B.D. Franks. 2007. *Fitness professional's handbook*, 5th ed. (Champaign, IL: Human Kinetics).

Montoye, H.J., T. Ayen, and R.A. Washburn. 1986. The estimation of $\dot{V}O_2$max from maximal and sub-maximal measurements in males, age 10-39. *Research Quarterly for Exercise and Sport* 57: 250-53.

Saltin, B., and P.-O. Åstrand. 1967. Maximal oxygen uptake in athletes. *Journal of Applied Physiology* 23: 353-58.

Evaluating Muscular Strength and Endurance

flexibility ? strength
- isolated small muscle groups vs. large groups

Purpose

This lab provides experience in administering muscular strength and endurance assessments. The lab focuses on easily administered tests: one-repetition maximum (1RM) for bench press (upper body strength), 1RM for seated leg press (lower body strength), 1 min curl-up (crunch) for endurance, 1 min push-up for endurance, and grip strength.

Materials

- Stopwatch or clock with a second hand
- Exercise mat
- Hand dynamometer
- Bench press and seated leg press equipment
- One copy of the Muscular Fitness Data Collection Worksheet (appendix B, page 128)

Background Information

Muscular strength and endurance are very important components of fitness. **Muscular strength** is the ability to exert maximal force in a single muscular contraction, whereas **muscular endurance** is the ability to exert a submaximal force repeatedly or over an extended period of time. Each of these components plays a unique role in activities of daily living and quality of life. Activities such as opening a jar, lifting a milk jug from a grocery cart, or opening a heavy door all require muscular strength. Conversely, activities such as sweeping a floor, hammering a nail, and sawing a board all require a great degree of muscular endurance. Through testing and evaluation you may be able to identify weaknesses in strength and endurance that may need improvement. Evaluating these components also enables you to determine the most appropriate course of action to improve a person's specific needs.

The Principle of Specificity

Training programs that emphasize exertion of force against a high resistance for a small number of repetitions enhance gains in strength, muscle size, and to a lesser extent, endurance. These programs are appropriate for people who are already reasonably healthy and fit. Programs that emphasize a relatively low resistance and a high number of repetitions enhance muscular endurance and to a smaller degree, strength and are more suited to clients or patients who are significantly unfit. These examples illustrate the principle of **specificity of training**. Keep this principle in mind when administering strength tests. If participants are following an isotonic training program, they should be tested with isotonic strength tests to assess isotonic strength changes. The mode of testing should also be appropriate to the subject population being tested. For example, when you are assessing an older population with no previous weightlifting experience, a hand dynamometer test to assess upper body strength is more appropriate than a 1RM bench press test.

Definitions

Following is a list of terms and definitions that are often used when discussing muscular strength and endurance.

- **isokinetic training**—Training that has both variable resistance and a speed-governing feature. Because isokinetic equipment controls the rate of contraction, it can potentially train the different types of muscle fiber.

- **isometric contraction**—A static muscle contraction wherein the overall length of the muscle does not change during the application of force against a fixed object.

- **isotonic contraction**—A dynamic muscle contraction in which the force remains constant. Isotonic exercises are typically performed with free weights or machines in which the resistance is "steered' along a fixed path. Accommodating resistance training (e.g., Nautilus, Cybex, etc.) is considered isotonic, although resistance is variable so that the lifter must exert maximum effort throughout the full range of motion.

- **muscular endurance**—The ability of a muscle to exert a submaximal force over a length of time.

- **muscular strength**—The maximum amount of force that can be exerted by a muscle in a single maximal effort.

- **Valsalva maneuver**—Increased pressure in the abdominal and thoracic cavities caused by breath holding and extreme effort (Howley and Franks 2007). Performing a Valsalva maneuver can inhibit the return of blood to the heart and increase blood pressure.

Procedures

1. Organize stations so that each lab group and student has an opportunity to participate in each assessment.

2. The following assessment procedures for one male and one female participant are required:

  a. One-repetition maximum (1RM) test for bench press: upper body strength

   b. One-repetition maximum (1RM) test for leg press: lower body strength

   c. One-minute curl-up test: abdominal endurance

   d. One-minute push-up test: upper body endurance

   e. Hand dynamometer test: hand strength

3. Record the participant's weight, age, and test data on the **Muscular Fitness Data Collection Worksheet**. Follow the specific test procedures for assessing muscular fitness that follow.

4. Use tables 8.1-8.5 to calculate percentiles and ratings for each participant.

5. The participant should not invoke the Valsalva maneuver during any of these exercises and should exhale during the concentric contraction phase during the bench press, leg press, pushup, and curl-up tests.

Table 8.1 Standard Values for One-Repetition Maximum for Bench Press

Percentile	<20	20-29	30-39	40-49	50-59	60+	Rating
	Age (yr)						
Men							
99	>1.76	>1.63	>1.35	>1.20	>1.05	>0.94	Superior
95	1.76	1.63	1.35	1.2	1.05	0.94	
90	1.46	1.48	1.24	1.1	0.97	0.89	Excellent
85	1.38	1.37	1.17	1.04	0.93	0.84	
80	1.34	1.32	1.12	1.0	0.9	0.82	
75	1.29	1.26	1.08	0.96	0.87	0.79	Good
70	1.24	1.22	1.04	0.93	0.84	0.77	
65	1.23	1.18	1.01	0.9	0.81	0.74	
60	1.19	1.14	0.98	0.88	0.79	0.72	
55	1.16	1.1	0.96	0.86	0.77	0.7	Fair
50	1.13	1.06	0.93	0.84	0.75	0.68	
45	1.1	1.03	0.9	0.82	0.73	0.67	
40	1.06	0.99	0.88	0.8	0.71	0.66	
35	1.01	0.96	0.86	0.78	0.7	0.65	Poor
30	0.96	0.93	0.83	0.76	0.68	0.63	
25	0.93	0.9	0.81	0.74	0.66	0.6	
20	0.89	0.88	0.78	0.72	0.63	0.57	
15	0.86	0.84	0.75	0.69	0.6	0.56	Very Poor
10	0.81	0.8	0.71	0.65	0.57	0.53	
5	0.76	0.72	0.65	0.59	0.53	0.49	
1	<.76	<.72	<.65	<.59	<.53	<.49	

(continued)

Table 8.1 *(continued)*

Percentile	<20	20-29	30-39	40-49	50-59	60+	Rating
			Age (yr)				
			Women				
99	>0.88	>1.01	>0.82	>0.77	>0.68	>0.72	Superior
95	0.88	1.01	0.82	0.77	0.68	0.72	
90	0.83	0.9	0.76	0.71	0.61	0.64	Excellent
85	0.81	0.83	0.72	0.66	0.57	0.59	
80	0.77	0.8	0.7	0.62	0.55	0.54	
75	0.76	0.77	0.65	0.6	0.53	0.53	Good
70	0.74	0.74	0.63	0.57	0.52	0.51	
65	0.7	0.72	0.62	0.55	0.5	0.48	
60	0.65	0.7	0.6	0.54	0.48	0.47	
55	0.64	0.68	0.58	0.53	0.47	0.46	Fair
50	0.63	0.65	0.57	0.52	0.46	0.45	
45	0.6	0.63	0.55	0.51	0.45	0.44	
40	0.58	0.59	0.53	0.5	0.44	0.43	
35	0.57	0.58	0.52	0.48	0.43	0.41	Poor
30	0.56	0.56	0.51	0.47	0.42	0.4	
25	0.55	0.56	0.51	0.47	0.42	0.4	
20	0.53	0.51	0.47	0.43	0.39	0.38	
15	0.52	0.5	0.45	0.42	0.38	0.36	Very Poor
10	0.5	0.48	0.42	0.38	0.37	0.33	
5	0.41	0.44	0.39	0.35	0.31	0.26	
1	<0.41	<0.44	<0.39	<0.35	<0.31	<0.26	

Bench press weight ratio = weight pushed/body weight

One-Repetition Maximum Test for Bench Press and Leg Press

The 1RM tests assess upper body strength (bench press) and lower body strength (leg press). Although the exercises are different, the steps for each are the same:

1. After a warm-up and familiarization with equipment, start with relatively low weight that the participant can easily and safely lift.
2. Add weight gradually until the participant can perform the lift correctly one time.
3. Encourage the participant to breathe freely with each lift.
4. Have the participant attempt to reach max within five trials with appropriate recovery, resting 1 to 2 min between trials (ACSM 2010a).

Table 8.2 Standard Values for One-Repetition Maximum for Leg Press

Percentile rankings* for men	Age					
	20-29	30-39	40-49	50-59	60+	
90	2.27	2.07	1.92	1.80	1.73	
80	2.13	1.93	1.82	1.71	1.62	
70	2.05	1.85	1.74	1.64	1.56	
60	1.97	1.77	1.68	1.58	1.49	
50	1.91	1.71	1.62	1.52	1.43	
40	1.83	1.65	1.57	1.46	1.38	
30	1.74	1.59	1.51	1.39	1.30	
20	1.63	1.52	1.44	1.32	1.25	
10	1.51	1.43	1.35	1.22	1.16	
Percentile rankings* for women	**Age**					
	20-29	30-39	40-49	50-59	60-69	70+
90	2.05	1.73	1.63	1.51	1.40	1.27
80	1.66	1.50	1.46	1.30	1.25	1.12
70	1.42	1.47	1.35	1.24	1.18	1.10
60	1.36	1.32	1.26	1.18	1.15	0.95
50	1.32	1.26	1.19	1.09	1.08	0.89
40	1.25	1.21	1.12	1.03	1.04	0.83
30	1.23	1.16	1.03	0.95	0.98	0.82
20	1.13	1.09	0.94	0.86	0.94	0.79
10	1.02	0.94	0.76	0.75	0.84	0.75

*Descriptors for percentile rankings: 70 = above average; 50 = average; 30 = below average; 10 = well below average.

Data for women provided by the Women's Exercise Research Center, The George Washington University Medical Center, Washington, D.C., 1998.

Data for men provided by The Cooper Institute for Aerobics Research, *The Physical Fitness Specialist Manual*, The Cooper Institute, Dallas, TX, 2005.

Reprinted, by permission, from V. Heyward, 2010, *Advanced fitness assessment and exercise prescription.* 6th ed. (Champaign, IL: Human Kinetics), 137.

One-Minute Curl-Up Test

1. The participant should assume a supine position on the floor with the knees bent so that the heels are positioned approximately 18 in. (7 cm) from the buttocks.

2. While the participant holds the arms at the sides, place a strip of masking tape on the floor at the fingertips. Place a second strip of tape exactly 8 cm (age ≥ 45 yr) or 12 cm (age < 45 yr) beyond the first strip (toward the participant's heels).

3. The participant does slow, controlled curl-ups lifting the shoulder blades off the mat and returning to the start position after each repetition. To successfully complete a repetition, the participant should touch the fingertips to the second strip of masking tape; the trunk should make a 30° angle with the mat and the low back should flatten before each curl-up.

4. Remind the participant to be sure to keep the neck straight; curving the neck can cause injury.

Table 8.3 Standard Values for One-Minute Partial Curl-Up

	Age (yr)					
	15-19	20-29	30-39	40-49	50-59	60-69
Men						
Excellent	25	25	25	25	25	25
Very good	23-24	21-24	18-24	18-24	17-24	16-24
Good	21-22	16-20	15-17	13-17	11-16	11-15
Fair	16-20	11-15	11-14	6-12	8-10	6-10
Needs improvement	≤15	≤10	≤10	≤5	≤7	≤5
Women						
Excellent	25	25	25	25	25	25
Very good	22-24	18-24	19-24	19-24	19-24	17-24
Good	17-21	14-17	10-18	11-18	10-18	8-16
Fair	12-16	5-13	6-9	4-10	6-9	3-7
Needs improvement	≤11	≤4	≤5	≤3	≤5	≤2

Source: *The Canadian Physical Activity, Fitness & Lifestyle Approach: CSEP-Health & Fitness Program's Health-Related Appraisal and Counseling Strategy*, 3rd Edition © 2003.

5. At the "go" signal from you, the participant perform as many curl-ups as possible in 1 min.

6. Score the test as the number of correctly performed curl-ups completed in the 1 min allotted (ACSM 2010a).

One-Minute Push-Up Test

1. Male participants perform this test in the standard position (on toes) and females in the modified position (on knees).

2. The participant must lower the body until the chin touches the mat. The abdomen should not touch the mat.

3. Remind the participant to keep the back straight at all times and to push up to a straight-arm position.

4. Score this test as the maximum number of push-ups performed consecutively without rest (Golding, Myers, and Sinning 1991).

Hand Dynamometer Test

1. To ensure a firm grasp on the instrument, the test participant should chalk or dry the hands before the test.

2. The participant holds the handgrip between the palm at the base of the thumb and the second joint of the fingers.

3. The participant holds the **dynamometer** out in front of the body and is allowed to move the body when actually squeezing.

4. The participant should squeeze the dynamometer with maximum effort.

5. Perform two trials with the participant using the dominant hand, with 1 to 2 min of rest between trials. Record the better of the trials for comparison to norms (Montoye and Lamphier 1977).

Table 8.4 Standard Values for One-Minute Push-Up

	Age (yr)					
	15-19	**20-29**	**30-39**	**40-49**	**50-59**	**60-69**
Men						
Excellent	≥39	≥36	≥30	≥25	≥21	≥18
Very good	29-38	29-35	22-29	17-24	13-20	11-17
Good	23-28	22-28	17-21	13-16	10-12	8-10
Fair	18-22	17-21	12-16	10-12	7-9	5-7
Needs improvement	≤17	≤16	≤11	≤9	≤6	≤4
Women						
Excellent	≥33	≥30	≥27	≥24	≥21	≥17
Very good	25-32	21-29	20-26	15-23	11-20	12-16
Good	18-24	15-20	13-19	11-14	7-10	5-11
Fair	12-17	10-14	8-12	5-10	2-6	2-4
Needs improvement	≤11	≤9	≤7	≤4	≤1	≤1

Source: *The Canadian Physical Activity, Fitness & Lifestyle Approach: CSEP-Health & Fitness Program's Health-Related Appraisal and Counseling Strategy*, 3rd Edition © 2003.

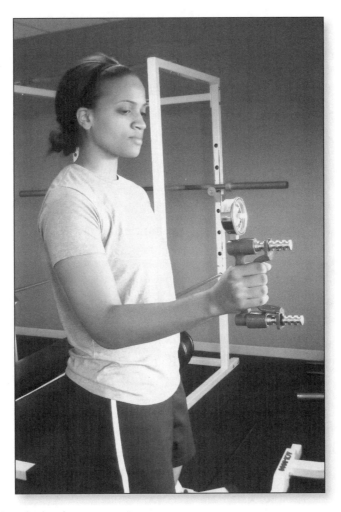

Figure 8.1 Handgrip dynamometer.

Table 8.5 Standard Values for Hand Strength

Percentile	Rating	Age (yr)				
		20-29	30-39	40-49	50-59	60 +
Men						
90	Well above average	>54	>53	>51	>49	>49
70	Above average	51-54	50-53	48-51	46-49	46-49
50	Average	43-50	43-49	41-47	39-45	39-45
30	Below average	39-42	39-42	37-40	35-38	35-38
10	Well below average	<39	<39	<37	<35	<35
Women						
90	Well above average	>36	>36	>35	>33	>33
70	Above average	33-36	34-36	33-35	31-33	31-33
50	Average	26-32	28-33	27-32	25-30	25-30
30	Below average	22-25	25-27	24-26	22-24	22-24
10	Well below average	<22	<25	<24	<22	<22

Hand strength values are expressed in kg, and should be tested on the dominant hand.

ICOSS, FITNESS HEALTH AND WORK CAPACITY, 1st Edition, © 1974, Pg. 61. Reprinted by permission of Pearson Education, Inc., Upper Saddle River, NJ.

Discussion Questions

1. Why is it important to choose the appropriate type of assessment technique?
2. Describe isokinetic strength and endurance training and the type of equipment it requires.
3. What is the level of strength and endurance of the participants on whom you have collected data? Do these participants need to improve in any areas? If yes, describe them.
4. What are the benefits and drawbacks of the grip dynamometer test?
5. Why do fitness professionals often examine abdominal endurance?

References

ACSM (American College of Sports Medicine). 2010a. *ACSM's guidelines for exercise testing and prescription.* 8th ed. Baltimore: Lippincott Williams & Wilkins.

ACSM (American College of Sports Medicine). 2010b. *Resource manual for guidelines for exercise testing and prescription.* 6th ed. Baltimore: Lippincott Williams & Wilkins.

Golding, J.A., C.R. Myers, and W.E. Sinning. 1991. *The Y's way to fitness.* Chicago: National Board of YMCA.

Howley, E.T., and B.D. Franks. 2007. *Fitness professional's handbook.* 5th ed. Champaign, IL: Human Kinetics.

Montoye, H.J. and D.K. Lamphier. 1977. Grip and arm strength in males and females age 10-59. *Research Quarterly for Exercise Science and Sport* 48: 109.

Evaluating Flexibility

Purpose

This lab presents six tests for evaluating flexibility: ankle flexibility test, shoulder elevation test, trunk extension test, sit-and-reach test, Thomas test, and straight-leg-raise test.

Materials

- Goniometer
- Sit-and-reach box
- Yardstick or meter stick
- Three copies of the Flexibility Data Collection Worksheet (appendix B, page 130)
- Mat or table

Background Information

Flexibility is the ability to move the body parts through a wide range of motion without undue strain to the articulations and muscle attachments. Maintaining a reasonable degree of flexibility is necessary for efficient body movement. Being flexible may also decrease the chances of sustaining muscle injury or soreness and low back pain. Proper muscle balance, in which agonist and antagonist muscle pairs maintain appropriate ratios of strength, flexibility, and length to one another, is important for avoiding musculoskeletal injury. Flexibility assessment and exercises are crucial for lengthening muscles that are too tight.

Muscle Injury and Soreness

To move body segments, the muscles opposite those performing the movement (antagonist muscles) must lengthen sufficiently. Tight muscles, tendons, and ligaments limit lengthening of the antagonist muscles and thus reduce the range of movement of body segments. Soreness or injury may result when tight muscles are subjected to strenuous physical activity.

Low Back Pain

Low back pain is one of the most common complaints among adults in the United States. Low back problems

- account for more lost work hours than any other type of occupational injury, and
- are the most frequent cause of activity limitation in people under 45 yr of age in the United States.

Muscular deficiencies, including lack of abdominal strength, have been recognized as important considerations in physical medicine regimens to treat back pain. The abdominal muscles play a major role in preventing excessive anterior or forward tilt of the pelvis, and strong abdominal musculature appears to play a very important role in supporting the trunk in postures often considered compromising to the low back. In forward-leaning postures, strong abdominal muscle contraction can appreciably increase intra-abdominal pressure; this appears to create a splinting-like effect on the trunk, which in turn decreases the stress placed on intervertebral discs.

Two groups of antagonist muscles (the hip flexors and the hip extensors) are also associated with low back pain; the former tilts the pelvis anteriorly and the latter tilts the pelvis posteriorly. Here the concern is lack of extensibility or too much tightness in the pelvis rather than lack of strength. Extreme shortening of either group can have a deleterious effect on the functioning of the low back (Howley and Franks 2007).

Measuring Flexibility

Flexibility measurements include flexion and extension movements. No general test is available that provides representative values of total body flexibility; tests are specific to each joint and muscle group and area of connective tissue. Because flexibility is joint specific, determining the range of motion of a few joints does not necessarily provide an indicator of flexibility in other joints.

The most accurate tests of flexibility are those in which a goniometer is used to measure the actual degrees of rotation of the various joints. A **goniometer** is a protractor type of instrument used to measure the joint angle at both extremes in the total range of movement. The double armed goniometer has two arms that attach to two body parts, with the center (fulcrum) of the instrument over the exact center of the joint tested (ACSM 2010b). The arms are aligned along the long axis of the bones of the adjacent segments (figure 9.1). It can be challenging to maintain the arms of the goniometer along the bones of the segment, however, this is critical to the reliability and validity of the assessment. In addition, it is important to isolate the joint movement by stabilizing the body while moving the joint.

Because hip flexors and hip extensors play a critical role in supporting a person's posture and avoiding low back discomfort, assessing flexibility of these muscle groups is important. Therefore, included are two simple tests that can provide information about the flexibility of these muscle groups.

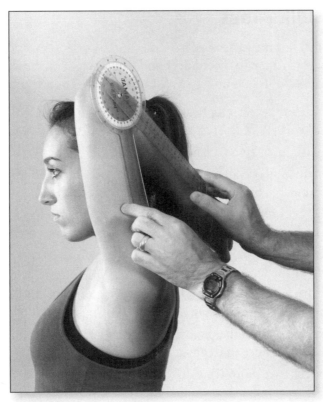

Figure 9.1   Double armed goniometer.

Procedures for Flexibility Tests

1. Organize stations so that each lab group and student has an opportunity to participate in each assessment.

2. The following assessment procedures for one male and one female participant are required:

   a. Ankle flexibility test

   b. Shoulder elevation test

   c. Trunk extension test

   d. Sit-and-reach test

   e. Thomas test

   f. Straight-leg-raise test

3. Record your results on the **Flexibility Data Collection Worksheet**. Follow the specific flexibility assessment procedures that follow.

4. Use tables 9.1 to 9.4 to calculate percentiles and ratings for each participant.

Ankle Flexibility Test

The ankle flexibility test measures a person's ability to flex and extend the ankle. Ankle inflexibility may contribute to discomfort and injuries associated with activities that use the lower leg, including running, walking, cycling, and swimming.

1. In preparation for the test, emphasize a brief warm-up of gradual ankle movements to increase the safety of the test and give the highest measurements possible.
2. Have the participant remove shoes.
3. The participant sits on a flat surface; the back of the knee touches the surface. The tester crouches or sits at the participant's side.
4. Keeping the heel on the ground, the participant pulls the foot in toward the body (dorsiflexed) as much as possible, keeping the toes straight (figure 9.1).
5. Measure this angle by aligning a protractor or goniometer with the anklebone and the side of the leg. Record this angle.
6. Then have the participant extend the foot (plantar flex) in the other direction as far as possible. Record the angle of this foot position.
7. The difference between the positions of dorsiflexion and plantar flexion is the average flexibility score in degrees of movement.
8. Repeat the test two more times (ACSM 2010b). Record the best score on the worksheet.
9. Using table 9.1, identify the percentile and rating for the ankle flexibility score in degrees of movement.

Shoulder Elevation Test

This test assesses the flexibility of the muscles in the front of the chest and shoulders (pectorals and anterior deltoids). Inflexibility in the chest and shoulders may limit

Table 9.1 Standard Values for Ankle Flexibility

Percentile	Rating	Ankle flexibility score*
Men		
90	Well above average	77-99
70	Above average	63-76
50	Average	48-62
30	Below average	34-47
10	Well below average	15-33
Women		
90	Well above average	81-89
70	Above average	68-80
50	Average	56-67
30	Below average	43-55
10	Well below average	32-42

*Score in degrees of movement.

Adapted from Johnson and Nelson 1969.

range of motion while participating in activities that use the upper body, such as throwing or swimming. This may cause shoulder pain and injury to the shoulder.

1. The participant stands with arms relaxed and hands pronated (knuckles facing forward) and grasps a yardstick or meter stick in the hands across the front of the body.

2. The tester measures the arm length from the acromion process to the top of the stick (proximal edge) (figure 9.2a).

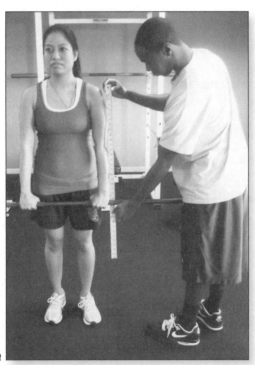

3. Next, the participant assumes a prone position lying on the floor with the chin touching the floor and the arms overhead, hands still holding the stick.

4. Have the participant slowly raise the stick as high as possible while keeping the chin on the floor and the elbows extended. Measure the distance in inches from the floor to the bottom of the stick (figure 9.2b). Repeat the test two more times.

5. To calculate flexibility, multiply the greatest height measured by 100 and divide this value by the arm length (ACSM 2010b).

6. Using table 9.2, identify the percentile and rating for the shoulder elevation score in inches.

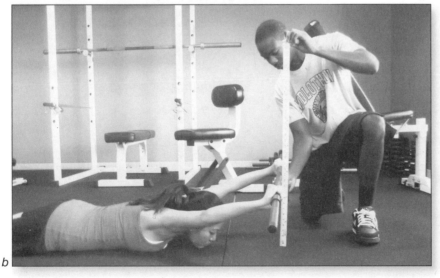

Figure 9.2 Be sure the participant's arms are relaxed and that the hands are pronated when you take the preliminary measurement for the shoulder extension test *(a)*. As the participant raises the arms, be sure that the elbows are extended and the chin remains in contact with the floor *(b)*.

Trunk Extension Test

This test assesses the flexibility of the muscles in the abdominal region. Flexibility and strength imbalances in the abdominal and lower back region are associated with back pain. This flexibility test assesses one's ability to extend the back while assessing the flexibility of the abdominal muscles.

Caution: People with existing or suspected back problems should not attempt this test because the motion involved exerts pressure on the posterior area of the lumbar vertebrae.

1. Make sure participants stretch before beginning the test.
2. First measure trunk length by having the participant sit back against a wall with legs extended out forward. Place the yardstick in front of the participant, between the legs, to make it easier to see the number for a more accurate reading. Trunk length is defined as the vertical distance (in.) between the floor and the suprasternal notch.
3. After taking this measurement, have the participant lie prone (on the stomach) and place the hands on the lower back.
4. A second person holds the participant's feet and hips to the floor while the participant slowly hyperextends the back as far up and back as possible.
5. The tester records the vertical distance (in.) between the mat and the suprasternal notch (figure 9.3).
6. Repeat the test two more times.
7. To calculate trunk extension, multiply the greatest distance measured by 100 and divide this value by the trunk length.
8. Using table 9.3, identify the percentile and rating for the trunk extension score.

Table 9.2 Standard Values for Shoulder Elevation

Percentile	Rating	Shoulder elevation score*
Men		
90	Well above average	106-123
70	Above average	88-105
50	Average	70-87
30	Below average	53-69
10	Well below average	35-52
Women		
90	Well above average	105-123
70	Above average	86-104
50	Average	68-85
30	Below average	50-67
10	Well below average	31-49

*Score in inches.

Adapted from Johnson and Nelson 1969.

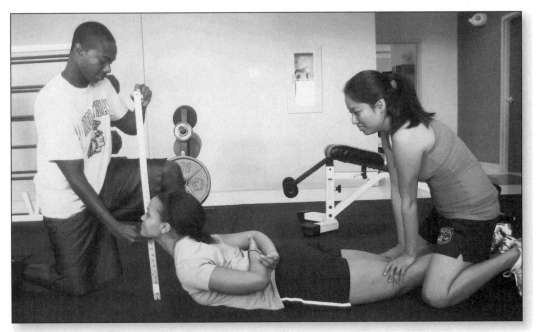

Figure 9.3 Trunk extension technique.

Table 9.3 Standard Values for Trunk Extension

Percentile	Rating	Trunk extension score*
Men		
90	Well above average	50-64
70	Above average	43-49
50	Average	37-42
30	Below average	31-36
10	Well below average	28-30
Women		
90	Well above average	48-63
70	Above average	42-47
50	Average	35-41
30	Below average	29-34
10	Well below average	23-28

*Score in inches.

Adapted from Johnson and Nelson 1969.

Sit-and-Reach Test

This test assesses the flexibility of the low back and hip joint. This test, although limited in its ability to predict low back pain, does assess primarily hamstring flexibility. Furthermore, because hamstring flexibility is imperative for activities of daily living and sport performance, this test is vital in health-related fitness testing.

Caution: To avoid the potentially negative effects of blood flow limitations to the heart and increases in blood pressure, the participant should not invoke the **Valsalva maneuver** and should breathe easily during the exercise.

1. The participant should perform a short warm-up before you administer this test. It is also recommended that the participant avoid fast, jerky movements, which may increase the possibility of injury.

2. Have the participant remove shoes.

3. Place a yardstick on the floor and apply tape across it at a right angle to the 15-in. mark. The participant sits with the yardstick between the legs, with legs extended at right angles to the taped line on the floor. Heels should touch the edge of the taped line and be about 10-12 in. apart.

4. If a standard sit-and-reach box is available, have the participant place the heels against the edge of the box.

5. The participant slowly reaches forward as far as possible with both hands on the yardstick, holding this position momentarily. Be sure that the participant keeps the hands parallel and does not stretch or lead with one hand. The fingertips of one hand can overlap those of the other, and the hands should be in contact with the yardstick or measuring portion of the sit-and-reach box (see figure 9.4).

6. Suggest that the participant exhale and drop the head between the arms when reaching. The tester should make sure the participant keeps the knees straight; however, do not press them down (ACSM 2010b).

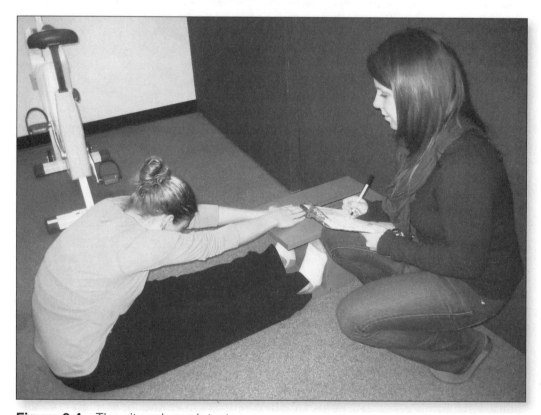

Figure 9.4 The sit-and-reach test.

7. The score is the most distant point (in in.) that the fingertips reach on the yardstick.
8. Repeat the test two more times and record the best of three trials.
9. Using table 9.4, identify the percentile and rating for the sit-and-reach score.

Thomas Test

The Thomas test assesses the flexibility of the hip flexors. These muscles tilt the pelvis anteriorly. An imbalance between these muscle and the hip extensors can negatively affect the functioning of the lower-back.

1. Have the participant lie supine (on the back).
2. The participant brings one leg (the contralateral leg, or the leg that is not being tested) in the direction of the chest just to the point where the lumbar spine is snug to the floor or table.
3. If the tested leg remains in contact with the floor or table during this maneuver, the hip flexors of that leg are adequately flexible.
4. If the tested leg rises, its hip flexors are likely to be inflexible (short) (Howley and Franks 2007).
5. Record whether the hip flexors in the right and left legs are flexible or inflexible.

Table 9.4 Standard Values for Trunk Flexion

Percentile	Rating	Trunk flexion score by age group*				
		20-29 yrs.	30-39 yrs.	40-49 yrs.	50-59 yrs.	60+ yrs.
Men						
90	Well above average	>21	>20	>19	>18	>17
70	Above average	19-21	18-20	17-19	16-18	15-17
50	Average	13-18	12-17	11-16	10-15	9-14
30	Below average	10-12	9-11	8-10	7-9	6-8
10	Well below average	<10	<9	<8	<7	<6
Women						
90	Well above average	>23	>22	>21	>20	>19
70	Above average	22-23	21-22	20-21	19-20	18-19
50	Average	16-21	15-20	14-19	13-18	12-17
30	Below average	13-15	12-14	11-13	10-12	9-11
10	Well below average	<13	<12	<11	<10	<9

*Score in inches.

Based on Golding Myers, and Sinning 1989.

Straight-Leg-Raise Test

The straight-leg-raise test assesses the flexibility of the hip extensors. These muscles tilt the pelvis posteriorly. An imbalance between these muscle and the hip flexors can negatively affect the functioning of the lower-back.

1. Have the participant lie supine (on the back).
2. Be sure the low back is snug against the floor or table (posteriorly rotated).
3. The tester raises one of the participant's legs while ensuring that the other leg remains extended and flat on the floor or table.
4. Measure the angle of flexion (range of motion) with one of the following:
   - A goniometer, by placing its axis on the greater trochanter
   - An inclinometer, placed just below the tibial tubercle
5. A minimum angle of 80° is acceptable for this passive straight-leg raise.
6. An angle of 90° is desirable (Howley and Franks 2007) .
7. Record the angle and report whether the range of motion is acceptable or unacceptable.

Discussion Questions

1. Compare the results of the three classmates you tested against the norms.
2. Summarize the six flexibility tests done in this lab. Can they be used to evaluate overall flexibility? Why or why not?
3. How is flexibility or lack of flexibility related to low back pain?
4. What can you do to improve the flexibility of your clients (i.e., what specific exercises can you recommend)?

Bibliography

ACSM (American College of Sports Medicine). 2010a. *ACSM's guidelines for exercise testing and prescription.* 8th ed. Baltimore: Lippincott Williams & Wilkins.

ACSM (American College of Sports Medicine). 2010b. *ACSM's Resource manual for guidelines for exercise testing and prescription.* 6th ed. Baltimore: Lippincott Williams & Wilkins.

Howley, E.T. and B.D. Franks. 2007. *Fitness professional's handbook*, 5th ed. (Champaign, IL: Human Kinetics).

ECG Placement and Monitor Operations

Purpose

This lab provides experience in locating, preparing, and placing the 10 electrodes used in a 12-lead electrocardiogram (ECG) and it describes the operations of the monitor, which you will use.

Materials

- Protective gloves
- Gauze and alcohol prep pads
- Dry-shave razors
- Electrodes
- Towel(s)
- Laundry bag
- Disinfectant soap
- Biohazard waste bag
- Biohazard sharps bag
- 10% bleach solution
- Voltmeter
- ECG monitor with paper
- Lab coat
- Scissors

Background Information

Electrocardiography is the science of monitoring the electrical function of the heart. The machine used to determine function is called an **electrocardiograph**, which records an **electrocardiogram (ECG).** An ECG is an electrical record of the current flowing through the heart muscle during the depolarization and repolarization of a contraction (Dubin 2000).

The ECG monitor will provide you with a real-time presentation of the electrical activity in the heart and a hard copy for record keeping. Various models of ECG monitors and electrocardiographs have unique features. Thus, to complete this lab it is imperative that you become familiar with the features of your ECG equipment.

The paper grid on the ECG (see figure 10.1) provides for a determination of duration of time (horizontal measurement); small block equals .04 sec; large block equals .20 sec. The 3 sec markers, of course, indicate 3 sec of elapsed time. The paper grid also provides for a determination of amplitude or voltage (vertical measure). This measurement is made in millimeters (mm); each small box represents 1 mm on the vertical axis above or below the isoelectric line (baseline; no electrical activity).

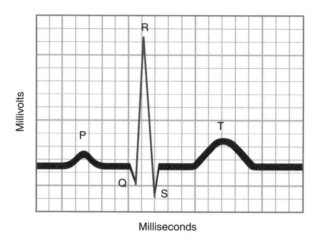

Figure 10.1 Annotated ECG printout.

Procedures

Following are the overall instructions for this lab along with the step-by-step procedures for ECG preparation and placement.

1. Obtain a lab coat and properly fitting protective gloves.
2. Set out the equipment needed to prepare the subject for the ECG.
3. Give the participant verbal instructions:

"My name is _____; I will be preparing you for an ECG."

"I will have to shave a few areas on the chest and rough up the area in order for the electrodes to have a good contact surface for adherence."

"The electrodes are necessary so that we can monitor the electrical activity of the heart during the test."

"A good contact surface will augment the monitor's ability to pick up the heart rate and also prevent the electrodes from falling off during the testing procedures."

"The rubbing with the gauze may cause some mild skin irritation, but this should subside within two days."

"Do you have any questions?"

4. Locate, prepare, and place electrodes on your lab partner (see Steps for ECG Preparation and Placement on page 79).

5. Locate electrode placements on at least three other lab partners for additional practice locating electrode placements. Many idiosyncrasies in body type can make locating the appropriate placement challenging. There is no need to prepare and place. The identification of placement is the most important learning experience.

6. Prepare the monitor.

   - Turn on the power for the electrocardiograph.
   - Turn on the power to the monitor, if necessary.
   - Be sure that the cable from the electrodes is connected into electrocardiograph.
   - The electrodes are not attached to the participant, thus the electrocardiograph should not be reading electrical activity.
   - Check the ECG paper supply. Be sure that you have enough paper for at least one test (minimum of 20 pages).
   - Be sure that the paper is set into the machine appropriately by pressing the Auto Run button. The paper should run smoothly and stop at the end of the page.
   - Make sure the paper speed is set to 25 mm/sec.

7. After placing the electrodes and preparing the monitor, place the label leads from the ECG on the appropriate electrodes.

   - Have the participant lie supine on the prep table with the left side closer to the technician.
   - The participant should lie still with arms at sides and legs uncrossed.
   - If the electrocardiograph includes a connection box for the electrodes, place this connection box on the participant's abdomen.
   - Begin placing the labeled electrodes on the corresponding electrode sites on the chest.

8. Be sure that you can monitor every lead without **artifact** (irrelevant or unwanted information) by examining the ECG on the monitor.

   - Press the button for leads I, II, and III. Examine the monitor for clear representation of the P-QRS-T complex.
   - Press the button for leads AVR, AVL, and AVF. Examine the monitor for clear representation of the P-QRS-T complex.
   - Press the button for leads V1, V2, and V3. Examine the monitor for clear representation of the P-QRS-T complex.
   - Press the button for leads V4, V5, and V6. Examine the monitor for clear representation of the P-QRS-T complex.
   - If artifact is present, it may be necessary to check and replace the lead that is displaying artifact.

- If everything is in order, have the participant lie still with no muscular movement.

9. Record an ECG.

   - Press the AUTO RUN button, which will automatically record an ECG for all 12 leads.
   - Be sure that the participant's name appears at the top of the ECG printout. If not, write in the space provided the participant's name and the condition (i.e., supine).

10. When the test period is over, press the button/key that will disconnect the electrical communication from the electrodes to the electrocardiograph, then remove the wires and electrodes from the participant.

11. Turn off the power on the monitor and the electrocardiograph.

12. Follow proper cleanup procedures.

    - Make sure all gauze and alcohol pads are discarded in the biohazard waste bags.
    - Make certain the dry-shave razor is properly discarded in the biohazard sharps container.
    - Spray the 10% bleach solution on the prep table after completing testing of each participant, and discard the towel in the laundry basket.
    - Remove the latex gloves and discard them in the biohazard waste bag.
    - Wash your hands with disinfectant soap after completing testing of each participant.

13. Calculate HR for each ECG in your group.

    - The electrical activity of the heart is represented on an ECG by a series of up-and-down deflections, or waves. The labels given to each deflection correspond to the letters P, Q, R, S, and T. One heartbeat on an ECG is represented by the P-QRS-T complex. The QRS represents the depolarization of the ventricles. Count the number of QRS complexes in a 6 sec period (two sequential 3 sec periods using the 3 sec marks) and multiply by 10.
    - The following numbers represent the calculated HR when two sequential R peaks are 1 small box (.4 sec), 2 small boxes, or 3 small boxes apart in distance: 300, 150, and 100, respectively. Furthermore, the calculated HR for when two sequential R peaks are 4 small boxes, 5 small boxes, and 6 small boxes apart in distance is 75, 60, and 50, respectively. This is referred to as the *triplicate technique for determining HR*.
    - Count the number of tiny boxes between two successive R peaks and divide by 1,500.

STEPS FOR ECG PREPARATION AND PLACEMENT

Following are the technician instructions for ECG preparation.

1. Have the participant lie supine on the prep table with the left side of the chest nearest the technician.

2. Mark the 10 areas (4 limb leads and 6 chest leads) to be shaved (see figure 10.2).

3. Note the following:
   - Never place an ECG electrode on a bony area; otherwise the monitor will pick up artifact, potentially resulting in irregular ECG recordings.
   - Begin shaving the areas for electrode placement on the limb lead areas first.
   - Use discretion with female clients. Explain exactly what you will be doing to the client before you do it. Be sure to maintain a professional approach and atmosphere.
   - Use a long stroke with the dry-shave razor.
   - If the subject has a lot of hair, it is acceptable to trim the hair first with scissors.
   - It may be necessary to dip the razor in a small container of water to rid the blades of excess hair.
   - Place the used dry-shave razor in the biohazard sharps container.

4. Shave the correct anatomical places.
   - Shave the locations for the right arm (RA) and left arm (LA) leads in the hollow space below the clavicle and the medial edge of the shoulder.
   - Shave the right leg (RL) and left leg (LL) lead locations approximately 1 in. above the navel below the rib cage on each side of the trunk.
   - From the clavicle, count down with your fingers to the fourth intercostal.
   - At this point, shave the V1 and V2 places (refer to figure 10.2).
   - The next space to be shaved on the chest is V4, which is to be placed directly below the nipple (mid clavicular) in the fifth intercostal space. Do not place the electrode on breast tissue. If the placement must be moved from the specified location, this should be reported on the ECG strip.
   - Then shave V3, midway between V2 and V4.
   - V6 is the next space to be shaved, in the midaxillary region under the left arm in the fifth intercostal space and horizontal to V4.
   - Finally, shave V5, placed midway between V4 and V6 (anterior axillary) (ACSM 2010a, 2010b).

5. Rub all the shaved areas with gauze and alcohol.
   - Either soak the gauze with alcohol and rub, thus roughing up and cleansing the area simultaneously, or rub the area with plain gauze to rough it up and then apply an alcohol prep pad to cleanse it.
   - The rubbed and cleansed area will be visibly red or pink.
   - Place the gauze and alcohol prep pads in the biohazard waste bag.
   - Follow the same directions for preparing the six chest lead sites.

6. Place the limb lead electrodes on the chest first. The limb leads will allow the technicians to view the heart through leads I, II, III, AVR, AVL, and AVF (Dubin 2000).

7. Next, place the chest lead electrodes on the chest.

8. Use the voltmeter to determine the conductivity of the electrode.
   - Place the black probe on the ground electrode (RL) and move the red probe around to the other electrodes.
   - Look for voltmeter readings of 600 MOhm or higher.
   - If the voltmeter readings are too low, it may be necessary to reapply the electrode after additional rubbing and cleansing of the area.

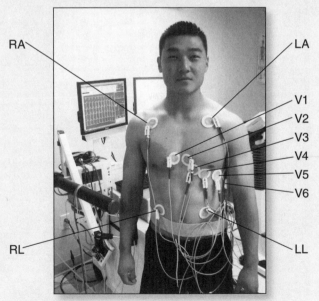

Figure 10.2 The 10 locations for electrode placement.

Discussion Questions

1. What are the basic dimensions and characteristics on the paper grid used for an ECG? Describe the horizontal and vertical measurements that can be taken.

2. Describe the basic components of the cardiac cycle as it is represented on an ECG.

3. Describe the 10 locations for the electrodes on a standard 12-lead electrocardiograph.

References

ACSM (American College of Sports Medicine). 2010a. *ACSM's guidelines for exercise testing and prescription*. 8th ed. Baltimore: Lippincott Williams & Wilkins.

ACSM (American College of Sports Medicine). 2010b. *ACSM's resource manual for guidelines for exercise testing and prescription*. 6th ed. Baltimore: Lippincott Williams & Wilkins.

Dubin, D. 2000. *Rapid interpretation of EKGs*. 6th ed. Tampa, FL: Cover.

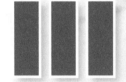

PART

III

Exercise Prescription

Part III focuses on exercise prescription. Lab 11 addresses the calculation of metabolic work for use in exercise prescription. Labs 12 and 13 focus on the three phases of exercise prescription (initial, improvement, and maintenance), assessment of the participant's goals, and gaining the participant's commitment to the exercise prescription. Finally, lab 14 challenges you to apply the techniques and principles presented in this manual by developing case studies. This process is facilitated by the worksheets and forms used in earlier labs. The forms are in appendix A and the worksheets are in appendix B. Remember to photocopy them for use in the labs.

Metabolic Calculations

Purpose

This lab demonstrates the knowledge and skill required to determine $\dot{V}O_2$ levels at given workloads in relative and absolute measures, MET levels, and kcal expenditure.

Materials

- Calculator
- Problems 1 to 10 (pages 85-87)
- Metabolic equations in appendix E
- %HRR and %$\dot{V}O_2$R Calculation Worksheet (appendix B, page 132)

Background Information

Metabolic equations serve two purposes for exercise professionals. The first is to calculate oxygen consumption, which allows you to determine caloric expenditure for a specific activity and duration. The second enables you to determine a target workload specific to the individual's goals and needs.

You can use several methods to determine target workload intensity for exercise prescription. The American College of Sports Medicine (ACSM 2010) recommends using %$\dot{V}O_2$ **reserve** (%$\dot{V}O_2$R) instead of %$\dot{V}O_2$. This is because Swain and Leutholtz (1997) demonstrated that %$\dot{V}O_2$R corresponds with % HR reserve (%HRR) more closely than does a direct percentage of $\dot{V}O_2$max. HRR accounts for the effect of varying resting HR levels from one person to the next and the impact of resting HR (RHR) on determining exercise intensity. To calculate %HRR and %$\dot{V}O_2$R, the resting measure of these variables (RHR and 3.5 ml/kg/min, respectively) is subtracted from the maximal levels of these variables, then the target percentage is calculated from this difference, and finally the resting measure is added back. **The %HRR and the %$\dot{V}O_2$R Calculations Worksheet** presents these steps clearly. The prescribed range of intensities of exercise for %HRR and %$\dot{V}O_2$R (40-85%) is discussed in lab 12.

Procedures

Solve the following problems. You may use a calculator, if necessary. You may find appendix D, Metric Conversions (pages 143), helpful as you complete this lab. See appendix F (page 149) for the answer key. We have walked you through the solution to a sample problem in the following box.

EXAMPLE PROBLEM

Paul Go is walking on a treadmill at 4.3 mph at a 6% grade for 30 min. His current body weight is 168 lb. He has a resting heart rate of 74 bpm. Calculate the following:

a. Relative $\dot{V}O_2$ in ml/kg/min

b. Absolute $\dot{V}O_2$ in L/min

c. MET level

d. Kilocalories per minute

e. Total caloric expenditure

EXAMPLE ANSWER CALCULATIONS

a. Relative $\dot{V}O_2$ in ml/kg/min

First, convert his speed from mph to m/min by multiplying 4.3 mph by 26.8, arriving at

115.24 m/min. Next, plug the converted information into the appropriate formula (see appendix E, page 145). Note that even though Paul is walking, due to his speed the appropriate formula to use for calculating his relative $\dot{V}O_2$ is the running formula.

$$\dot{V}O_2 = 0.2 \text{ (speed)} + 0.9 \text{ (speed)(fractional grade)} + 3.5 \text{ ml/kg/min}$$

$$\dot{V}O_2 = 0.2 \times 115.24 + 0.9 \text{ (115.24} \times .06) + 3.5 \text{ ml/kg/min}$$

$$\dot{V}O_2 = 23.05 + 6.22 + 3.5 \text{ ml/kg/min}$$

$$\dot{V}O_2 = 32.77 \text{ ml/kg/min}$$

b. Absolute $\dot{V}O_2$ in L/min

First, convert Paul's body weight from lb to kg by dividing his weight by 2.2 (or multiplying his weight by 0.454), arriving at 76 kg.

Next, now that you have Paul's relative $\dot{V}O_2$ from part a, you can find his absolute $\dot{V}O_2$ by multiplying 32.77 ml/kg/min by his body weight in kg and then dividing by 1,000.

$$a \dot{V}O_2 = r \dot{V}O_2 \text{ ml/kg/min} \times \text{wt (kg)} \div 1,000$$

$$a \dot{V}O_2 = 32.77 \text{ ml/kg/min} \times 76 \text{ kg} \div 1000$$

$$a \dot{V}O_2 = 2.49 \text{ L/min}$$

c. MET level

To find Paul's MET level, simply divide his relative $\dot{V}O_2$ by 3.5 ml/kg/min.

METs = r $\dot{V}O_2$ ÷ 3.5 ml/kg/min

METs = 32.77 ml/kg/min ÷ 3.5 ml/kg/min

METs = 9.36

d. Kilocalories per minute

You have determined that Paul's a $\dot{V}O_2$ is 2.49 L/min. By multiplying this by 5, you will determine how many kilocalories he is expending per minute while exercising.

kcal/min = a $\dot{V}O_2$ × 5

kcal/min = 2.49 L/min × 5

kcal/min = 12.45

e. Total caloric expenditure

Paul is expending 12.45 kcal/min while he is exercising. To find his total caloric expenditure, simply multiply his kcal/min by the number of minutes he exercised.

Total kcal = kcal/min × total minutes

Total kcal = 12.45 × 30

Total kcal = 373.5

PROBLEM 1

Rahul Singh is running on a treadmill at 6.5 mph at a 5% grade for 45 min. His current body weight is 176 lb. Calculate the following:

a. Relative $\dot{V}O_2$ in ml/kg/min
b. Absolute $\dot{V}O_2$ in L/min
c. MET level
d. Kilocalories per minute
e. Total caloric expenditure

PROBLEM 2

Elias Fernandez is running on a treadmill at 6.4 mph at a 3% grade for 40 min. His current body weight is 182 lb. Calculate the following:

a. Relative $\dot{V}O_2$ in ml/kg/min
b. Absolute $\dot{V}O_2$ in L/min
c. MET level
d. Kilocalories per minute
e. Total caloric expenditure

From E. Acevedo and M. Starks, 2011, *Exercise testing and prescription lab manual,* 2nd ed. (Champaign, IL: Human Kinetics).

PROBLEM 3

Brandon Williamson is walking on a treadmill at 3.5 mph for 30 minutes. His current bodyweight is 187 lb. His absolute $\dot{V}O_2$ level at this intensity is 2.3 L/min. Calculate the following:

a. Relative $\dot{V}O_2$ in ml/kg/min
b. MET Level
c. The grade of the treadmill
d. Kilocalories per minute
e. Total caloric expenditure

PROBLEM 4

Susan Lin Yan steps on a 15-inch step at 30 steps/min for 30 min. Her current body weight is 125 lbs. Calculate the following:

a. Relative $\dot{V}O_2$ in ml/kg/min
b. Absolute $\dot{V}O_2$ in L/min
c. MET level
d. Kilocalories per minute
e. Total caloric expenditure

PROBLEM 5

Bill Shadle's maximum workload while riding a Monark cycle ergometer at 60 rpm is 4 kg of resistance. His body weight is 195 lb. He cycled for 45 min. Calculate the following:

a. Relative $\dot{V}O_2$ in ml/kg/min
b. Absolute $\dot{V}O_2$ in L/min
c. MET level
d. Kilocalories per minute
e. Total caloric expenditure

PROBLEM 6

Michelle Dloughy weighs 118 lb and is walking up and down an 8-inch step at 30 steps/min for 30 min. Calculate the following:

a. Relative $\dot{V}O_2$ in ml/kg/min
b. Absolute $\dot{V}O_2$ in L/min
c. MET level
d. Kilocalories per minute
e. Total caloric expenditure

From E. Acevedo and M. Starks, 2011, *Exercise testing and prescription lab manual*, 2nd ed. (Champaign, IL: Human Kinetics).

PROBLEM 7

At maximal effort Amiir Abduljaber is running on a treadmill at 6.0 mph up a 12% grade. His current body weight is 168 lb. Calculate the following:

a. Relative $\dot{V}O_2$ in ml/kg/min
b. Absolute $\dot{V}O_2$ in L/min
c. MET level
d. Kilocalories per minute
e. Determine target $\dot{V}O_2$ at 75% $\dot{V}O_2R$

PROBLEM 8

Tumoni Johnson is walking on a treadmill at 3.7 mph for 60 min. Her current body weight is 124 lb. Her current functioning $\dot{V}O_2$ level is 1.1 L/min. Calculate the following:

a. Kcal/min
b. Total caloric expenditure
c. Relative $\dot{V}O_2$ in ml/kg/min
d. Met Level
e. Grade of the treadmill

PROBLEM 9

Lynn Aaron is cranking a Monark arm ergometer at 50 rpm with a resistance of 2.5 kg. This is her maximum workload. Her current body weight is 126 lb. Calculate the following:

a. Relative $\dot{V}O_2$ in ml/kg/min
b. Absolute $\dot{V}O_2$ in L/min
c. MET level
d. Kilocalories per minute
e. Target $\dot{V}O_2$ at 80% $\dot{V}O_2R$

PROBLEM 10

Richard K. Williams is running on a treadmill at a certain speed with a grade of 5% at 44.67 ml/kg/min for 30 min. His body weight is 215 lb. Calculate the following:

a. Absolute $\dot{V}O_2$ in L/min
b. The speed of the treadmill
c. MET level
d. Kilocalories per minute
e. Total caloric expenditure

From E. Acevedo and M. Starks, 2011, *Exercise testing and prescription lab manual,* 2nd ed. (Champaign, IL: Human Kinetics).

References

ACSM (American College of Sports Medicine). 2010. *ACSM'S guidelines for exercise testing and prescription.* 8th ed. Baltimore: Lippincott Williams & Wilkins.

Swain, D.P., and B.C. Leutholtz. 2002. *Exercise prescription: a case study approach to the ACSM Guidelines.* Champaign, IL: Human Kinetics.

Assessing Participant Goals and Gaining Commitment to Physical Activity

Purpose

This lab facilitates exercise prescription and adherence by demonstrating how to assess a participant's fitness and health goals. As physical adaptations occur and fitness is improved, fitness and health goals may also change. Thus, assessment follows a series of cyclical steps:

1. Assessment of health-related fitness
2. Modification of behavior (developing an exercise prescription to achieve goals)
3. Monitoring behavior (exercise journals, record keeping)
4. Periodic reevaluation of health-related fitness, modification of behavior (if necessary), and continual monitoring of behavior (Griffin 2006)

Materials

Two copies each of the following forms:

- Exercise Prescription Interview Form (appendix A, page 112)
- Fitness Goals and Exercise Prescription Form (appendix A, page 113)
- Fitness Contract (appendix A, page 114)
- Resistance Exercise Journal (appendix A, page 115)
- Cardiovascular Exercise Journal (appendix A, page 116)
- Fitness Assessment Form With Exercise Prescription Guidelines (appendix A, page 110)

Background Information

Four steps of client motivation are integral to developing an effective exercise prescription.

1. Assessment of health-related fitness

   - Interview the client to assess his or her health-related fitness goals (**Exercise Prescription Interview Form**).
   - As you initiate a relationship with a client, it is important to present and conduct yourself in a professionally appropriate manner.
   - In addition, effective motivators who enhance adherence most often have a positive rapport with clients.
   - This can be important for maintaining open communication.

2. Modification of behavior

   - The aim is to develop an exercise prescription to achieve goals.
   - Establish goals that include a clear strategy for achieving each goal. (**Fitness Goals and Exercise Prescription Form**)
     - The goals should be challenging and attainable.
     - Each goal must be desirable to the client.
     - There should be both short-term and long-term goals.
     - Goals should be highly specific and practical.
     - The client must believe that the exercise prescription created to achieve the goal will be effective.
     - The client must believe that the exercise prescription is achievable.
   - With the client, fill in the "Exercise prescription" areas of the Fitness Goals and Exercise Prescription Form using the guidelines from the client's **Fitness Assessment Form With Exercise Prescription Guidelines** that address each goal.
   - Guide the client in examining and addressing both environmental support for and barriers to implementing the prescription strategies for each goal.
   - Have the client rate importance, commitment, and confidence for reaching each goal. This is likely to illuminate motivation issues that you may want to address (Griffin 2006).
   - Behavioral contracts (**Fitness Contract**) can be used to demonstrate and document commitment to the fitness program.

3. Monitoring of behavior

   - This can be done through exercise journals and record keeping.
   - Clients should keep a clear daily record of the behaviors that are part of the goal strategies.

4. Periodic reevaluation

- Health-related fitness should continue to be the focus.
- Modification of behavior may be necessary when life events impact exercise behavior.
- Monitoring behavior can ensure that the client is continually aware of his or her exercise behaviors.

Procedures

1. Complete one set of the forms for yourself (see appendix A, pages 110-116). You need to fill out only one week in the **Resistance Exercise Journal** and **Cardiovascular Exercise Journal.**

2. Find one other person outside of class and take him or her through the process of completing the second set of forms. This person needs to complete the exercise journals for only one week.

Discussion Questions

1. What are some important characteristics of a professional in the fitness promotion field?

2. How can an exercise specialist build rapport with a client?

3. What are factors to consider when setting goals? What should be included in a complete goal-setting program?

4. In setting goals, how might a client address expected barriers to an exercise program?

5. How would you handle a client who is having difficulty following the proposed strategy for achieving his or her goal?

6. Would you expect that goals might change as the client ages, achieves certain goals, or has a change in daily schedule? How would you handle a situation in which a client does not want to change his or her goals?

Bibliography

ACSM (American College of Sports Medicine). 2010. *ACSM's guidelines for exercise testing and prescription.* 8th ed. Baltimore: Lippincott Williams & Wilkins.

Griffin, J.C. 2006. *Client-centered exercise prescription.* 2nd ed. Champaign, IL: Human Kinetics.

Prescriptions for Initial Conditioning, Improvement, and Maintenance

Purpose

This lab presents and describes the general principles of exercise prescription. You will learn to integrate fitness assessment results into useful information for prescribing exercise for clients.

Materials

- One copy of the Fitness Assessment Form With Exercise Prescription Guidelines (appendix A, page 110)
- Three copies of the %HRR and %$\dot{V}O_2$R Calculation Worksheet (appendix B, page 132)

Background Information

The ACSM guidelines for exercise prescription are based on evidence for the specific stimulus necessary to cause adaptations to the cardiovascular and musculoskeletal systems. These adaptations are based on the principles of overload (repeated exposure, including appropriate rest, to unaccustomed load is associated with adaptation of improved functional capacity), specificity (adaptations are specific to stimulus and systems involved), and progression (improved functioning requires increases in stimulus to cause further adaptation) (ACSM 2010). Furthermore, the guidelines for caloric expenditure are supported with evidence demonstrating the impact of caloric expenditure on weight loss and body composition (United States Department of Health and Human Services 1996).

Training Session Components

Each training session should contain three components; warm-up phase, stimulus (exercise) phase, and cool-down phase. These phases are important in allowing the body's systems to prepare for activity and recover appropriately from activity. Most important, the cardiovascular system adapts to meet oxygen requirements of the activity, while the musculoskeletal system adapts to facilitate movement by reducing the viscosity of joint lubricants. These adaptations may reduce the likelihood of injury. With regard to the four major components of health-related fitness, the warm-up phase or the cool-down phase can include musculoskeletal flexibility. The stimulus or exercise phase can be either a cardiorespiratory stress or a skeletal muscle stress, with energy expenditure being calculated for aerobic activity.

The ACSM exercise prescription guidelines are presented in the **Fitness Assessment Form With Exercise Prescription Guidelines.** These guidelines are intentionally broad and must be used with good clinical judgment based on the client's fitness level, health status, personal interests and goals, and age.

Cardiorespiratory Fitness

HR and $\dot{V}O_2$ maintain a positive linear relationship as workload increases. This relationship allows for the determination of exercise intensity through the calculation of percent HR reserve (%HRR; Karvonen equation) and percent $\dot{V}O_2$ reserve (%$\dot{V}O_2$R). These two methods provide reliable and relatively accurate measures of exercise intensity. Following are the equations for %HRR and %$\dot{V}O_2$R. If calculating exercise intensity from a straight percentage of HRmax you can expect that %$\dot{V}O_2$max will be 10 to 15% lower than the % HRmax. Note that RPE can be a useful tool in identifying a workload that is comfortable for the client. In particular, for clients who are taking a medication that can alter HR or those who have difficulty palpitating HR, RPE can be helpful in providing a cue for determining exercise intensity (ACSM 2010; Howley and Franks 2007; Pollack et al. 1998).

Percent Heart Rate Reserve

$$(\text{HRmax} - \text{resting HR}) \times \% \text{ intensity} + \text{resting HR} = \text{target HR}$$

Percent $\dot{V}O_2$ Reserve

$$(\dot{V}O_2\text{max} - \text{resting } \dot{V}O_2) \times \% \text{ intensity} + \text{resting } \dot{V}O_2 = \text{target } \dot{V}O_2$$

Energy Expenditure

The expenditure of energy can be of significant concern to those who are beginning an exercise program. A good understanding of how the body utilizes energy for physical activity can limit participants' unrealistic expectations about weight loss. Unrealistic expectations are likely to also impact motivation. The metabolic cost of a prescribed activity can be determined with the metabolic calculation presented in lab 11. Furthermore, this metabolic cost can be used to determine the caloric expenditure of that activity.

Following is an example of the calculations for a person who weighs 75 kg. Determining the caloric expenditure of running at 5 mph at 2% grade using metabolic calculations equals a $\dot{V}O_2$ of 32.61 ml/kg/min (which would be a target $\dot{V}O_2$).

32.61 ml/kg/min −3.50 ml/kg/min (subtract 1 MET to determine net caloric expenditure) = 29.11 ml/kg/min

29.11 ml/kg/min ×1,000 (to convert to L/kg/min) = .02911 L/kg/min

.02911 L/kg/min × 75 kg (to convert to L/min) = 2.18

2.18 L/min × 5 kcal/min (standard used for kcal expenditure for $\dot{V}O_2$ in L/min) = 10.9 kcal/min

10.9 kcal/min expended by this individual while running at 5 mph at 2% grade

If the goal is 1,000 kcal/wk, the client would have to accumulate 91.7 minutes of this activity throughout the week (1,000 kcal ÷ 10.9 kcal/min = 91.7). The client could achieve this caloric expenditure with approximately 30 minutes of this activity, 3 days a week.

Musculoskeletal Flexibility

Lack of flexibility in the lower back and posterior thigh regions seem to be associated with increased risk for development of chronic lower back pain. Furthermore, mainstreaming flexibility may facilitate elderly people's ability to perform activities of daily living. Proprioceptive neuromuscular facilitation (PNF) is not advised for use by anyone without specific knowledge of the techniques.

Muscular Fitness

People require some level of muscular strength and endurance to perform activities of daily living. Thus, maintaining muscular fitness is critical for maintaining functional independence throughout the life span and limiting musculoskeletal injury. It is important to avoid the Valsalva maneuver when lifting heavy weight; this is accomplished by expiring when moving the weight against gravity (concentric contraction) and inspiring when moving the weight with gravity (eccentric contraction).

Progression Through Exercise Prescription

Following are the guidelines for progressing through the three stages of an exercise program (ACSM 2010).

1. Initial conditioning stage
   - This stage should progress through 4 weeks.
   - Unfit inactive individuals start at 40 to 60 %HRR.
   - Each session lasts 15 to 20 minutes initially and progresses to 30 minutes.
   - Schedule 3 or 4 sessions a week (reevaluate goals; address whether goals should be adapted for any initial adaptations that may have occurred).

2. Improvement stage
   - This stage typically lasts between 4 and 5 months.
   - Periodically reassess fitness and reevaluate goals.
   - For most people, the target range for intensity should progress to 85 %HRR.

- Increase the duration every 2 to 3 weeks until the client can perform moderate-to-vigorous exercise continuously for 20 to 30 minutes.
- Schedule 3 to 5 sessions a week.
- Alter the strength training program to facilitate the adaptations necessary to meet goals.

3. Maintenance Stage

- This stage typically begins after 5 to 6 months, when the participant has reached preestablished fitness goals and is no longer interested in further increases in the conditioning stimulus.
- The client's focus should turn to meeting long-term goals (reassess fitness and reevaluate goals).
- The activities selected for this phase should be enjoyable and promote lifetime participation in physical activity.
- Reevaluate strength goals and alter the strength training program accordingly.

The exercise prescription for enhancing muscular fitness should increase in resistance as adaptations occur and goals are achieved. To maintain muscular fitness the client should perform at least 1 set of 8 to 10 different exercises, at least twice a week. Flexibility should be addressed throughout each stage. Following initial assessments, the prescription should focus on enhancing range of motion for the muscle groups that the client is using during the physical activity session and those that are determined to be limiting the client's range of motion. Following this initial adaptation, the prescription for flexibility should be directed toward addressing the client's goals and any limitation or misalignment that is diagnosed (Griffin 1998).

Procedures

1. Complete the **Fitness Assessment Form With Exercise Prescription Guidelines** for at least one person in the class.
2. From lab 11 (metabolic calculations) determine the caloric expenditure for three of the problems. Calculate the number of 30-minute workouts a week each of the three individuals in the problems would have to complete to expend 1,000 kcal.
3. Calculate %HRR for each of the three individuals.

Discussion Questions

1. What are some concerns to consider when prescribing resistance exercise?
2. As time progresses and the client is adapting to the exercise stress, what are some factors that you may want to address to maintain motivation and compliance?

References

ACSM (American College of Sports Medicine). 2010. *ACSM's guidelines for exercise testing and prescription.* 8th ed. Baltimore: Lippincott Williams, & Wilkins.

Griffin, J.C. 1998. *Client-centered exercise prescription.* Champaign, IL: Human Kinetics.

Howley, E.T., and B.D. Franks. 2007. *Fitness professional's handbook.* 5th ed. Champaign, IL: Human Kinetics.

Pollock, M.L., G.A. Gaesser, J.D. Butcher, et al. 1998. The recommended quantity and quality of exercise for developing and maintaining cardiorespiratory and muscular fitness, and flexibility in healthy adults. *Medicine and Science in Sports Exercise 30*: 975-991.

United States Department of Health and Human Services. 1996. *Physical activity and health: A report of the Surgeon General.* Washington, DC: International Medical Publishing.

Case Study Reports

Purpose

This lab provides an opportunity to develop case studies on a variety of fitness program participants.

Materials

- Case studies from lab 3
- Equipment for fitness testing
- Five copies of Medical History Form (appendix A, page 102) or its shorter alternative, the Health Screening Form (appendix A, page 105)
- Five copies of Informed Consent Form (appendix A, page 106)
- Five copies of Physician Release Form (appendix A, page 107)
- Five copies of Risk Stratification Form (appendix A, page 108)
- Five copies of Fitness Assessment Form With Exercise Prescription Guidelines (appendix A, page 110)
- Five copies of Exercise Prescription Interview Form (appendix A, page 112)
- Five copies of Fitness Goals and Exercise Prescription Form (appendix A, page 113)
- Five copies of Fitness Contract (appendix A, page 114)
- Copies of the corresponding worksheets to the data that you collected on your case studies

Background Information

Fitness professionals must formulate individualized exercise prescriptions as carefully as any other preventive or therapeutic intervention. As you develop an exercise prescription for each client, always remember the FITT principle (frequency, intensity, time, and type). Developing an adequate and safe exercise prescription also depends on the availability of the following information:

1. Sufficient medical information to assess the client's past and present health status, including patient demographics, a medical and surgical history, findings of physical examination, signs and symptoms, essential test results (blood chemistry, ECG, echocardiography, and angiography), and a risk factor assessment and profile

2. Graded exercise test data (if advised) that quantify current physical work capacity

3. Documentation of current exercise habits

4. The client's expression of interests, needs, and objectives for wanting to participate in an exercise training program

A case study is a concise report of the essential information pertaining to the risk status, exercise evaluation, or activity prescription of a given person. The following procedures are steps that can simplify the development of a case study using the forms presented throughout this manual.

Procedures

1. Review the case studies used in lab 3.

2. Create five new case studies and exercise prescriptions on five classmates or volunteers. Remember to include the following:

   a. **Medical History Form** or its shorter alternative, the **Health Screening Form**

   b. **Informed Consent Form**

   c. **Physician Release Form** (if necessary)

   d. Testing results and calculations

   e. **Risk Stratification Form**

   f. **Fitness Assessment Form With Exercise Prescription Guidelines**

   g. **Exercise Prescription Interview Form**

   h. **Fitness Goals and Exercise Prescription Form**

   i. **Fitness Contract**

3. Suggest any other appropriate preventive or therapeutic interventions.

Appendix A

Exercise Testing and Prescription Forms

Medical History Form

Participant's name: _____ Date: _____/_____/_____

Address: _____

Weight: _____ Height: _____ Age: _____ Date of birth: _____/_____/_____

Female ❑   Male ❑

Home phone: (_____) _____   Business phone: (_____) _____

In case of emergency contact: _____

Contact's phone: (_____) _____

Name of personal physician: _____

Physician's phone: (_____) _____

Date and reason last consulted: _____

1. Please place a check mark beside those conditions that you currently have or have had in the past.

   _____ heart attack   _____ thrombophlebitis   _____ 5 to 19 lbs overweight

   _____ angina   _____ asthma   _____ high blood pressure

   _____ abnormal ECG   _____ fixed-rate pacemaker   _____ low blood pressure

   _____ heart medications   _____ embolism   _____ diabetes

   _____ valve disease   _____ respiratory infections _____ epilepsy

   _____ aneurysm   _____ irregular heartbeats   _____ anemia

   _____ 20 lb or more overweight

2. Has your physician ever advised you against exercise? _____Yes _____No

   If yes, why? _____

   _____

   _____

3. Do you currently have or have you had any of the following conditions?

   _____ arthritis   _____ ankle/foot injury   _____ shoulder/clavicle injury

   _____ low back pain   _____ arm/elbow injury   _____ knee/thigh injury

   _____ calcium deposit   _____ nerve damage   _____ upper back injury

   _____ head/neck injury   _____ bone fracture   _____ wrist/hand injury

   _____ hip/pelvis injury   _____ tennis elbow

   If yes, please explain and include dates: _____

   _____

   _____

4. Are you currently receiving physical therapy? _____Yes _____ No

   If yes, therapist's name and phone number: _____

   _____ (_____)_____

5. May we call him/her? _____Yes _____ No

From E. Acevedo and M. Starks, 2011, *Exercise testing and prescription lab manual*, 2nd ed. (Champaign, IL: Human Kinetics).

Medical History Form *(continued)*

6. Do you have any conditions or past injuries that may limit the range of motion of your muscles, joints, bones, spinal column, or any other part of your body that may be aggravated by exercise? _____Yes _____ No

   If yes, please explain: _____
   _____
   _____

7. Are you currently taking any medications on a regular basis? _____Yes _____ No

   If yes, please list names and dosages of each: _____
   _____
   _____

8. Are you currently under a doctor's care? _____Yes _____ No

   If yes, please furnish his/her name and phone number: _____
   _____ (_____)_____

9. May we call him/her? _____Yes _____ No
10. What is your current weight? _____
11. What was your weight 1 year ago? _____ 5 years ago? _____ at age 20? _____
12. Are you currently on a specific diet? _____Yes _____ No

    If yes, please describe: _____
    _____
    _____

13. Are you tired or fatigued most of the day? _____Yes _____ No
14. Are you tired or fatigued at a specific time of the day? _____Yes _____ No

    If yes, when: _____
    _____
    _____

15. On the average, how many times per year do you travel extensively? _____
16. On the average, how many hours a day do you spend at work? _____
    How many days a week? _____
17. How would you rate the level of physical activity you perform while at work?
    _____ very inactive _____ inactive _____ moderate _____ active _____ very active
18. How would you rate the level of physical activity you perform during leisure time?
    _____ very inactive _____ inactive _____ moderate _____ active _____ very active
19. Are you presently performing any standard physical fitness program (e.g., aerobics)?
    _____Yes _____ No

If yes, please note how many times per week you exercise, the duration of exercise sessions (in min), and what types of activity you participate in (e.g., jogging, walking, lifting weights, etc.).

_____
_____
_____

From E. Acevedo and M. Starks, 2011, *Exercise testing and prescription lab manual*, 2nd ed. (Champaign, IL: Human Kinetics). *(continued)*

Medical History Form (continued)

20. How physically fit do you feel at present?

_____ unfit _____ less than fit _____ fit _____ more than fit _____ very fit

21. If the equipment and facilities were available, which physical activities would you be interested in learning about and participating in?

_____ hiking   _____ bicycling   _____ aerobics

_____ weightlifting   _____ swimming   _____ jogging

_____ handball   _____ calisthenics   _____ volleyball

_____ tennis   _____ badminton   _____ racquetball/squash

_____ golf   _____ yoga   _____ supervised conditioning

_____ sailing   _____ horseback riding

22. Do you have any exercise equipment or device at home? _____ Yes _____ No

If yes, specify: _____

_____

_____

23. Do you or did you participate in high school or college athletics? _____ Yes _____ No

If yes, specify: _____

_____

_____

24. Would any activities not interest you or possibly cause you discomfort or pain? _____ Yes _____ No

If yes, please specify: _____

_____

_____

25. What are your primary reasons for visiting _____ ?

(name of your facility)

_____ general conditioning   _____ swimming   _____ stress reduction

_____ muscular strength   _____ running   _____ socializing

_____ flexibility   _____ weight loss   _____ facility offerings

_____ cardiovascular conditioning

I have answered the preceding questions to the best of my ability. I have understood all the questions asked of me and have been given the opportunity to have any questions clarified to my satisfaction. I further understand that thorough and honest responses to these questions are essential to my safety, health, and wellness.

Signature _____ Date _____/_____/_____

Witness _____ Date _____/_____/_____

From E. Acevedo and M. Starks, 2011, *Exercise testing and prescription lab manual*, 2nd ed. (Champaign, IL: Human Kinetics).

Health Screening Form

Participant's name: _____ Date: _____/_____/_____

Weight: _____Height: _____Age: _____

Female ❑   Male ❑

This form is intended to obtain relevant information about your health that will assist the staff in helping you with your program. Please answer all questions to the best of your knowledge.

1. Weight

   How would you describe your current body weight?

   _____ Underweight (under ideal)   _____ 5 to 19 lb overweight

   _____ Normal   _____ More than 20 lb overweight

2. Blood pressure

   Do you have high blood pressure? _____ Yes _____ No

   Have you had high blood pressure in the past? _____ Yes _____ No

   Are you on medication for high blood pressure? _____ Yes _____ No

3. Smoking

   Do you smoke? _____ Yes _____ No

   Are you a former smoker? _____ Yes _____ No

   If yes, please give the date you quit. _____

4. Diabetes

   Do you have diabetes? _____ Yes _____ No

5. Heart problems

   Have you ever had a heart attack? _____ Yes _____ No

   Have you ever had heart surgery? _____ Yes _____ No

   Have you ever had angina? _____ Yes _____ No

6. Family history

   Have any of your blood relatives had heart disease, heart surgery, or angina?
   _____ Yes _____ No

7. Orthopedic problems

   Do you have any serious orthopedic problems that would prevent you from exercising?
   _____ Yes _____ No

   If yes, please explain:

   _____

   _____

8. Other problems

   Do you have any reason to believe you should not exercise? _____ Yes _____ No

   If yes, please explain:

   _____

   _____

9. Emergency

Please list a relative we may contact in case of an emergency:

Name: _____ Telephone: _____

Relation: _____

From E. Acevedo and M. Starks, 2011, *Exercise testing and prescription lab manual*, 2nd ed. (Champaign, IL: Human Kinetics).

Informed Consent Form

1. Purpose and Explanation of the Test

The test you will perform will be on a cycle ergometer. The test will begin with a low amount of effort and will increase gradually depending on your fitness level. This increase in effort will continue until you reach your target heart rate or symptoms such as fatigue, shortness of breath, or discomfort appear. At that point, the cycle ergometer will be slowed. It is important to understand that you may stop the test at any point if you are feeling fatigue or any other discomfort.

2. Attendant Risks and Discomforts

During the exercise test a possibility of adverse changes exists. The changes can include abnormal blood pressure, fainting, disorders of heart rhythm, and in very rare instances, heart attack. A preliminary examination and observations during testing will help to minimize risks. Emergency equipment and trained personnel are available to deal with complications.

3. Responsibilities of the Participant

Knowledge you have of previous medical conditions and current health status directly affects your safety during the exercise test. It is your responsibility to fully disclose any medical conditions or physical abnormalities you may have as well as medications recently taken. This includes any unusual feeling you may perceive during the test. It is extremely important that you communicate with the testing staff.

4. Benefits to Be Expected

The results obtained from this test will be used in the evaluation of your current health status and to determine the activities that are appropriate for you.

5. Inquiries

We encourage any questions about the procedures and results of the exercise test. If you have any further questions, please ask.

6. Use of Medical Records

All information obtained from this exercise test will be treated as confidential. It will not be released or revealed to any person without your express written consent. The information gathered may be used for statistical or scientific purposes with your right of privacy retained.

7. Freedom of Consent

I give my consent freely to engage in an exercise test to ascertain my exercise capacity as well as the condition of my cardiovascular health. My permission to perform this exercise test is given willingly. I understand that I am free to stop the test at any time if I so choose.

I have read this consent form and I understand it, and any questions which may have occurred to me have been answered to my satisfaction. I consent to participate in this test.

Signed: _____ Date: _____/_____/_____

_____   _____
Witness   Physician supervising test

From E. Acevedo and M. Starks, 2011, *Exercise testing and prescription lab manual*, 2nd ed. (Champaign, IL: Human Kinetics).

Physician Release Form

Dear Doctor _____,

_____ has applied for enrollment in the fitness testing
(name of applicant)

and\or exercise programs at _____.
(name of your facility)

The fitness testing program involves a submaximal test for cardiorespiratory fitness, body composition analysis, flexibility test, and muscular strength and endurance tests. The exercise programs are designed to start at an easy level and become progressively more difficult over time. All fitness tests and exercise programs will be administered by qualified personnel trained in conducting exercise tests and exercise programs.

Completing the following form does not mean that you assume any responsibility for our administration of the fitness testing and/or exercise programs. If you know of any medical or other reasons why the applicant's participation in the fitness testing and/or exercise programs would be unwise, please indicate it on this form.

Report of Physician

___ I know of no reason that the applicant may not participate.

___ I believe the applicant can participate, but I urge caution because of the following:

_____

_____

_____

___ The applicant should not engage in the following activities:

_____

_____

_____

___ I recommend that the applicant not participate.

Physician Signature: _____ Date: _____

Address _____ Telephone _____

City and State _____ Zip _____

Risk Stratification Form

Name: _____ Date: _____

Risk factors	Yes/No	Comments
Positive (Yes +1)		
Family history	_____	_____
Cigarette smoking	_____	_____
Hypertension	_____	_____
Hypercholesterolemia	_____	_____
Impaired fasting glucose	_____	_____
Obesity	_____	_____
Sedentary lifestyle	_____	_____
Negative (Yes −1)	_____	_____
High serum HDL cholesterol	_____	_____

Total risk factors _____

Major signs or symptoms suggestive of CVD or PVD (Yes +1)	Yes/No	Comments
Pain, discomfort in the chest (or other anginal equivalent), neck, jaw, arms, or other areas that may be due to ischemia	_____	_____
Shortness of breath at rest or with mild exertion	_____	_____
Dizziness or syncope	_____	_____
Orthopnea or paroxysmal	_____	_____
nocturnal dyspnea		
Palpitations or tachycardia	_____	_____
Intermittent claudication	_____	_____
Known heart murmur	_____	_____
Unusual fatigue or shortness of breath with usual activities	_____	_____

Total signs or symptoms _____

Initial risk stratification

Low risk _____   Moderate risk _____   High risk _____

Current medical examination before participation

Moderate exercise (circle one)	Not necessary	Not necessary	Recommended
Vigorous exercise (circle one)	Not necessary	Recommended	Recommended

Risk Stratification Form *(continued)*

Physician supervision of exercise test

Submaximal test (circle one)	Not necessary	Not necessary	Recommended
Maximal test (circle one)	Not necessary	Recommended	Recommended

Additional Medical Concerns

Medications: _____

_____

_____

_____

Orthopedic limitations: _____

_____

_____

_____

Other:

_____

_____

_____

_____

Note: For all **positive risk factors** that are answered **Yes,** add 1 in the space provided, and for all **negative risk factors** answered **Yes,** subtract 1 in the space provided. For all **signs or symptoms** answered **Yes,** add 1 to the space provided. Scores should be totaled and the individual stratified according to ACSM guidelines.

From E. Acevedo and M. Starks, 2011, *Exercise testing and prescription lab manual*, 2nd ed. (Champaign, IL: Human Kinetics).

Fitness Assessment Form
With Exercise Prescription Guidelines

Fitness Assessment Results	Fitness Level Classification		Exercise Prescription Guidelines
	Percentile	**Rating**	
Cardiorespiratory fitness			
$\dot{V}O_2$max: _____ ml/kg/min	_____	_____	**Mode:** Large muscle group for prolonged periods of activity
			Frequency: 3-5 days/week
			Intensity: 40-85% of %HRR or %$\dot{V}O_2$R; RPE of 12-16
			Duration: 20-30 min
Musculoskeletal flexibility			
Sit-and-reach: _____ in.	_____	_____	**Mode:** Static or proprioceptive neuromuscular facilitation (PNF)
Shoulder elevation: _____ in.	_____	_____	**Frequency:** 2-3 days/week
			Intensity: Position of mild discomfort
			Duration: 10-30 sec for static; 6 sec contraction followed by 10-30 sec of assisted stretch for PNF
			Repetitions: 3-4 for each stretch
Muscular fitness			
Upper body endurance: _____reps	_____	_____	**Mode:** Resistance training (8-10 exercises)
Abdominal endurance: _____reps	_____	_____	**Frequency:** 2-3 days/week
Upper body strength: _____1RM	_____	_____	**Intensity:** A resistance (weight) that will elicit volitional exhaustion within 8-12 reps for individuals less than 50 yr of age, and 10-15 reps for more frail or older individuals. 1-2 min between sets.
Leg strength: _____1RM	_____	_____	**Duration:** Each rep lasting approximately 2 sec for concentric and eccentric contractions (controlled manner)
	_____	_____	**Repetitions:** 8-12 reps for individuals less than 50 yr of age and 10-15 reps for more frail or older individuals

Fitness Assessment Form
With Exercise Prescription Guidelines *(continued)*

Fitness Assessment Results	Fitness Level Classification		Exercise Prescription Guidelines
	Percentile	Rating	
Energy expenditure			
Body fat: _____%	_____	_____	**Caloric threshold:** 1,000 kcal per week; 150-400 kcal per day.
Body mass index: _____kg/m²	_____ (classification)		
	_____ (classification)		
Waist circumference: _____cm			

From E. Acevedo and M. Starks, 2011, *Exercise testing and prescription lab manual*, 2nd ed. (Champaign, IL: Human Kinetics).

Exercise Prescription Interview Form

Before this interview, be sure that the client is informed of the benefits and importance of fitness, his or her specific health-related fitness assessment results, and the exercise prescription guidelines. The fitness assessment results and the exercise prescription guidelines are found on the **Fitness Assessment Form With Exercise Prescription Guidelines** (page 110). It is also important that the client be aware of the connection between choice of health-related behaviors and health fitness–related outcomes (e.g., improved overall health, enhanced fitness, decrease in morbidity and mortality).

Preferences and Interests Related to Fitness

What mode (type) of physical activity do you enjoy (e.g., walking, bicycling, jogging, swimming, doing yard work, etc.)?

_____

_____

_____

_____

Do you prefer group or individual training? What type of training environment do you prefer (e.g., outdoor, indoor, cold, hot, pool, etc.)?

_____

_____

_____

_____

Are there activities that you do not like and would like to avoid?

_____

_____

_____

_____

Would you like to do the same activities regularly, or would you prefer variety in your workout schedule?

_____

_____

_____

_____

Would you like more information or resources on particular activities or health-related information?

_____

_____

_____

_____

From E. Acevedo and M. Starks, 2011, *Exercise testing and prescription lab manual*, 2nd ed. (Champaign, IL: Human Kinetics).

Fitness Goals and Exercise Prescription Form

Be sure to set challenging, attainable, desirable, specific, and practical goals. The exercise prescription should also meet these criteria and follow the ACSM guidelines for exercise prescription. In your exercise prescription be sure to address factors that may be used to support you in reaching your goal and address possible hurdles/barriers that may deter you from reaching your goal. Be sure to rate how important reaching the goal is for you, how committed you are to the goal, and how confident you are in reaching the goal.

Fitness goal A: _____

Exercise prescription:

_____

_____

_____

_____

0	10	20	30	40	50	60	70	80	90	100

Low   *Moderate*   *High*

Importance   *Importance*   *Importance*

Commitment   *Commitment*   *Commitment*

Confidence   *Confidence*   *Confidence*

Importance score _____

Commitment score _____

Confidence score _____

Fitness goal B: _____

Exercise prescription:

_____

_____

_____

_____

0	10	20	30	40	50	60	70	80	90	100

Low   *Moderate*   *High*

Importance   *Importance*   *Importance*

Commitment   *Commitment*   *Commitment*

Confidence   *Confidence*   *Confidence*

Importance score _____

Commitment score _____

Confidence score _____

From E. Acevedo and M. Starks, 2011, *Exercise testing and prescription lab manual*, 2nd ed. (Champaign, IL: Human Kinetics).

Fitness Contract

This Fitness Contract is made and entered into by and between _____

and _____. This contract is subject to the following terms and conditions:

1. To the best of my abilities I will follow the strategies set forth within my Fitness Goals and Exercise Prescription.

2. To the best of my abilities I will document my fitness related behaviors in my Fitness Journal.

3. As time progresses, when necessary I will refresh my commitment by reading and reviewing information related to health behaviors and health outcomes.

4. I will reassess my fitness level within 6 weeks (__/__/__). At that time I will reevaluate my Fitness Goals and, if necessary, set new goals.

In witness whereof, the parties hereto have executed this Fitness Contract on this the _____

day of_____, 20___.

_____   _____
Fitness Client Signature   Fitness Consultant

From E. Acevedo and M. Starks, 2011, *Exercise testing and prescription lab manual*, 2nd ed. (Champaign, IL: Human Kinetics).

Resistance Exercise Journal

Name: _____

Exercise	Warm-up	Working set	%1RM	Date	Comments
	×	×			
	×	×			
	×	×			
	×	×			
	×	×			
	×	×			
	×	×			
	×	×			
	×	×			
	×	×			
	×	×			
	×	×			
	×	×			
	×	×			
	×	×			
	×	×			
	×	×			
	×	×			
	×	×			
	×	×			
	×	×			
	×	×			
	×	×			
	×	×			
	×	×			
	×	×			
	×	×			

From E. Acevedo and M. Starks, 2011, *Exercise testing and prescription lab manual*, 2nd ed. (Champaign, IL: Human Kinetics).

Cardiovascular Exercise Journal

Week _____

Date	Activities	Time of day	HR/RPE	Comments/Notes

Week _____

Date	Activities	Time of day	HR/RPE	Comments/Notes

From E. Acevedo and M. Starks, 2011, *Exercise testing and prescription lab manual*, 2nd ed. (Champaign, IL: Human Kinetics).

Appendix B

Data Collection Worksheets

Cycle Ergometer Calibration Worksheet

1. Make sure the bike is on a level surface.
2. Record the precalibration readings.
3. Adjust the plate to zero (no tension).
4. Calibrate the pendulum weight.
5. Record the calibrated readings.
6. Using a ruler or straightedge, complete each linearity graph.

Precalibration Readings

Measured weight (lb/kg)	Scale reading (lb/kg)

Calibrated Readings

Measured weight (lb/kg)	Scale reading (lb/kg)

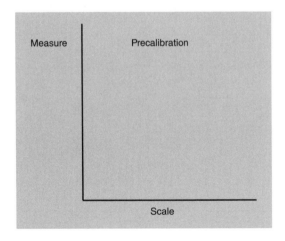

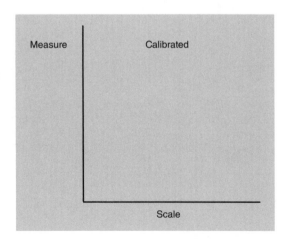

Sphygmomanometer Calibration Worksheet

1. Zero out the gauges (be sure they are set to zero).
2. Inflate the instruments.
3. Record the calibrated readings.
4. Complete the linearity graph.

Calibrated Readings

Mercury Gauge	Aneroid Gauge	Difference
200 mmHg		
180 mmHg		
160 mmHg		
140 mmHg		
120 mmHg		
100 mmHg		
80 mmHg		
60 mmHg		
40 mmHg		

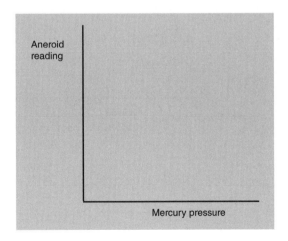

From E. Acevedo and M. Starks, 2011, *Exercise testing and prescription lab manual*, 2nd ed. (Champaign, IL: Human Kinetics).

Weight Scale Calibration Worksheet

1. Zero out the scale (be sure the weights are set to zero).
2. Place the varying weights on the scale.
3. Record the calibrated readings.
4. Complete the linearity graph.

Calibrated Readings

Measured weight (lb/kg)	Scale reading (lb/kg)

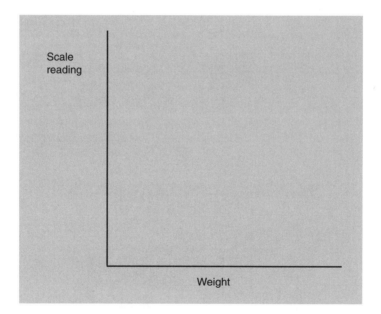

From E. Acevedo and M. Starks, 2011, *Exercise testing and prescription lab manual*, 2nd ed. (Champaign, IL: Human Kinetics).

Hanging Scale Calibration Worksheet

1. Disconnect the chair or harness.
2. Place the varying weights on the scale.
3. Record the calibrated readings.
4. Complete the linearity graph.

Calibrated Readings

Measured weight (lb/kg)	Scale reading (lb/kg)

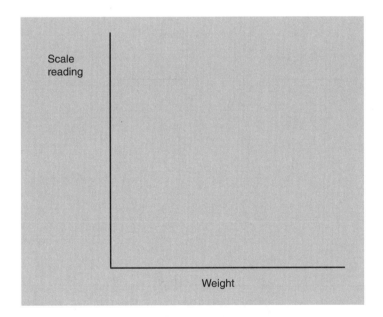

From E. Acevedo and M. Starks, 2011, *Exercise testing and prescription lab manual*, 2nd ed. (Champaign, IL: Human Kinetics).

measured by Christina

Skinfold and Circumference
Data Collection Worksheet

Participant's name: _Grace Fonte_   Date: _03/ 21/ 17_

Skinfold measurements (sites in duplicate, within 1-2 mm)		
Abdominal	_20_ + _16_ / 2 =	18 ∅
Biceps	_5_ + _6_ / 2 =	5.5
Chest	_5_ + _6_ / 2 =	5.5 ∅
Medial calf	_9_ + _8_ / 2 =	8.5
Midaxillary	_10_ + _7_ / 2 =	8.5 ∅
Subscapular	_11_ + _10_ / 2 =	10.5 ∅
Supraillium	_9_ + _8_ / 2 =	8.5 ∅
Thigh	_22_ + _21_ / 2 =	‑ 21.5 ∅
Triceps	_10_ + _12_ / 2 =	11 ∅
Circumferential measurements (sites in duplicate, within 1-2 mm)		
Waist	_92 97_ + _96 98_ / 2 =	91.5
Hip	_97_ + _98_ / 2 =	97.5

From E. Acevedo and M. Starks, 2011, *Exercise testing and prescription lab manual*, 2nd ed. (Champaign, IL: Human Kinetics).

Heart Rate and Blood Pressure
Data Collection Worksheet

Participant's name: _____ Date: _____/_____/_____

Normal BP range (if known): _____/_____

Resting HR Measurements

10-sec count	_____ × 6 = _____ bpm
15-sec count	_____ × 4 = _____ bpm
30-sec count	_____ × 2 = _____ bpm
60-sec count	_____ bpm

Resting BP Measurements

BP reading	_____ / _____
BP reading	_____ / _____
BP reading	_____ / _____

Exercise HR and BP Measurements

Stage	Resistance	Measurement start time	HR	BP	Comments
1	0.5 kg	1:45 2:00 2:45	_____ bpm _____ bpm	____/____	
2	1.0 kg	4:45 5:00 5:45	_____ bpm _____ bpm	____/____	
3	1.5 kg	7:45 8:00 8:45	_____ bpm _____ bpm	____/____	
4	2.0 kg	10:45 11:00 11:45	_____ bpm _____ bpm	____/____	
Recovery	0.5 kg	1:45 2:00 2:45	_____ bpm _____ bpm	____/____	

From E. Acevedo and M. Starks, 2011, *Exercise testing and prescription lab manual*, 2nd ed. (Champaign, IL: Human Kinetics).

Åstrand-Ryhming Data Collection Worksheet

Participant's name: _____ Date: _____/_____/_____

Weight: _____ Age: _____

Resting HR: _____ bpm   Resting BP: _____/_____

Stage	Resistance	Measurement start time	HR	BP	RPE/Comments
Testing	____ kp	0:45	_____ bpm		
		1:30		____/____	
		1:45	_____ bpm		
		2:45	_____ bpm		
		3:30		____/____	
		3:45	_____ bpm		
		4:45	_____ bpm		
		5:30		____/____	
		5:45	_____ bpm		
*Extra level (if necessary)	____ kp	6:30		____/____	
		6:45	_____ bpm		
Final HR	Average of fifth and sixth HRs*		_____ bpm		
Recovery	____ kp	1:00	_____ bpm	____/____	
		2:00	_____ bpm	____/____	
		3:00	_____ bpm	____/____	
		4:00	_____ bpm	____/____	

*Average of sixth and seventh if extra level is necessary.

From E. Acevedo and M. Starks, 2011, *Exercise testing and prescription lab manual*, 2nd ed. (Champaign, IL: Human Kinetics).

YMCA Test Data Collection Worksheet

Participant's name: __Grance Fonte__   Date: _03_ / _07_ / _2017_

Weight: __13 6__   Age: __22__

Resting HR: __61__ bpm   Resting BP: _103_ / _53_

Age-predicted HRmax: 220 – __22__ = __198__ bpm

Target HR: __168.3__ bpm (70 %HRR or 85% of age-predicted max)
_(85%)_

or __156.9 (70%)__

Stage	Resistance	Measurement start time	HR	BP	RPE/Comments
1	_150 kp (.5) kg_	1:45	91 bpm	141 / 129	8 (very light)
		2:30		/	
		2:45	174 bpm	154 / 101	
2	450 kp (1.5) kg	4:45	116 bpm	115 / 43	13 (somewhat hard)
		5:30		/	
		5:45	120 bpm	119 / 90	
3	300 kp (1.0) kg	7:45	128 bpm	141 / 80	9 (very light)
		8:30		/	
		8:45	89 bpm	135 / 62	
4	450 kp 1.5 kg	10:45	180 bpm	134 / 54	12 (fairly light)
		11:30		/	
		11:45	130 bpm	128 / 178	
Recovery	36 kp .5 kg	1:00	68 bpm	118 / 81	7 (very very light)
		2:00	117 bpm	115 / 59	
		3:00	163 bpm	99 / 35	
		4:00	86 bpm	109 / 48	

Seat height → 6 inches

ADHD students + exercise

anxious / angry kids go on bike
→ Brenda Smith
some information
use of activity in class?

student
2-3 die
– training environment

From E. Acevedo and M. Starks, 2011, *Exercise testing and prescription lab manual*, 2nd ed. (Champaign, IL: Human Kinetics).

BMI and Body Fatness Data Collection Worksheet

Participant's name: _____Grace Fonte_____ Date: _21_ / _03_ / _17_

BMI Calculation

Calculate BMI (wt/ht^2) in the space provided.

Weight: _58,5_ (kg) Height: _162_ ^{cm} (m)

BMI = _____ (wt) = _____ (ht^2)

Classification: _____ (from table 6.1)

Risk Classification

Hip circumference: _97,5_

Waist circumference: _91,5_

Waist-to-hip ratio: _____

Body Composition

Body density: _1,056_

Body density = _____ – _____ (sum of ___ skinfolds) + _____ (sum of ___ skinfolds) – _____ (___ yr)

% body fat: _____

$$\text{body fat} = \frac{\rule{3cm}{0.4pt}}{\text{body density}} - \rule{3cm}{0.4pt}$$

Percentile: _____ (from table 6.2)

Rating: _____ (from table 6.2)

Fat mass: _____

Lean mass: _____

From E. Acevedo and M. Starks, 2011, *Exercise testing and prescription lab manual*, 2nd ed. (Champaign, IL: Human Kinetics).

Muscular Fitness Data Collection Worksheet

One-Repetition Maximum (1RM) for Bench Press: Upper Body Strength

Male

Participant's name: _____

Date: _____/_____/_____

Weight: _____(lb) Age: _____

_____ 1RM ÷ _____Body weight = _____Ratio

Percentile: _____ Rating: _____
     (from table 8.1)   (from table 8.1)

Female

Participant's name: _____

Date: _____/_____/_____

Weight: _____(lb) Age: _____

_____ 1RM ÷ _____Body weight = _____Ratio

Percentile: _____ Rating: _____
     (from table 8.1)   (from table 8.1)

One-Repetition Maximum (1RM) for Leg Press: Lower Body Strength

Male

Participant's name: _____

Date: _____/_____/_____

Weight: _____(lb) Age: _____

_____ 1RM ÷ _____Body weight = _____Ratio

Percentile: _____ Rating: _____
     (from table 8.2)   (from table 8.2)

Female

Participant's name: _____

Date: _____/_____/_____

Weight: _____(lb) Age: _____

_____ 1RM ÷ _____Body weight = _____Ratio

Percentile: _____ Rating: _____
     (from table 8.2)   (from table 8.2)

One-Minute Curl-Up: Abdominal Endurance

Male

Participant's name: _____

Date: _____/_____/_____

Age: _____ # of reps: _____

Percentile: _____ Rating: _____
     (from table 8.3)   (from table 8.3)

Female

Participant's name: _____

Date: _____/_____/_____

Age: _____ # of reps: _____

Percentile: _____ Rating: _____
     (from table 8.3)   (from table 8.3)

(continued)

From E. Acevedo and M. Starks, 2011, *Exercise testing and prescription lab manual*, 2nd ed. (Champaign, IL: Human Kinetics).

Muscular Fitness Data Collection Worksheet (continued)

One-Minute Push-Up: Upper Body Endurance

Male

Participant's name: _____

Date: _____/_____/_____

Age: _____ # of reps: _____

Percentile: _____ Rating: _____
(from table 8.4)   (from table 8.4)

Female

Participant's name: _____

Date: _____/_____/_____

Age: _____ # of reps: _____

Percentile: _____ Rating: _____
(from table 8.4)   (from table 8.4)

Hand Dynamometer: Hand Strength

Male

Participant's name: _____

Date: _____/_____/_____

Age: _____ Dominant Hand L / R (circle one)

Trial 1: _____(kg) Trial 2: _____(kg)

Percentile: _____ Rating: _____
(from table 8.5)   (from table 8.5)

Female

Participant's name: _____

Date: _____/_____/_____

Age: _____ Dominant Hand L / R (circle one)

Trial 1: _____(kg) Trial 2: _____(kg)

Percentile: _____ Rating: _____
(from table 8.5)   (from table 8.5)

From E. Acevedo and M. Starks, 2011, *Exercise testing and prescription lab manual*, 2nd ed. (Champaign, IL: Human Kinetics).

Flexibility Data Collection Worksheet

Ankle Flexibility Test

Male

Participant's name: _____

Date: _____/_____/_____

Dorsiflexion ° trial 1:   _____

Dorsiflexion ° trial 2:   _____

Plantar flexion ° trial 1: _____

Plantar flexion ° trial 2: _____

    _____ degrees dorsiflexion of best trial

– _____ degrees plantar flexion of best trial

= _____ degrees flexibility

Percentile: _____ Rating: _____
       (from table 9.1)   (from table 9.1)

Female

Participant's name: _____

Date: _____/_____/_____

Dorsiflexion ° trial 1:   _____

Dorsiflexion ° trial 2:   _____

Plantar flexion ° trial 1: _____

Plantar flexion ° trial 2: _____

    _____ degrees dorsiflexion of best trial

– _____ degrees plantar flexion of best trial

= _____ degrees flexibility

Percentile: _____ Rating: _____
       (from table 9.1)   (from table 9.1)

Shoulder Elevation Test

Male

Participant's name: _____

Date: _____/_____/_____

Trial 1: _____ (in.)

Trial 2: _____ (in.)

Trial 3: _____ (in.)

    _____ best trial (in.) × 100

÷ _____ arm length (in.)

= _____ shoulder elevation score

Percentile: _____ Rating: _____
       (from table 9.2)   (from table 9.2)

Female

Participant's name: _____

Date: _____/_____/_____

Trial 1: _____ (in.)

Trial 2: _____ (in.)

Trial 3: _____ (in.)

    _____ best trial (in.) × 100

÷ _____ arm length (in.)

= _____ shoulder elevation score

Percentile: _____ Rating: _____
       (from table 9.2)   (from table 9.2)

(continued)

From E. Acevedo and M. Starks, 2011, *Exercise testing and prescription lab manual*, 2nd ed. (Champaign, IL: Human Kinetics).

Flexibility Data Collection Worksheet *(continued)*

Trunk Extension Test

Male

Participant's name: _____

Date: _____/_____/_____

Trial 1: _____ (in.)

Trial 2: _____ (in.)

Trial 3: _____ (in.)

_____ best trial (in.) × 100

÷ _____ trunk length (in.)

= _____ Trunk extension score

Percentile: _____ Rating: _____
(from table 9.3)   (from table 9.3)

Female

Participant's name: _____

Date: _____/_____/_____

Trial 1: _____ (in.)

Trial 2: _____ (in.)

Trial 3: _____ (in.)

_____ best trial (in.) × 100

÷ _____ trunk length (in.)

= _____ Trunk extension score

Percentile: _____ Rating: _____
(from table 9.3)   (from table 9.3)

Sit-and-Reach Test

Male

Participant's name: _____

Date: _____/_____/_____

Circle the best trial:

Trial 1: _____ (in.)

Trial 2: _____ (in.)

Trial 3: _____ (in.)

Percentile: _____ Rating: _____
(from table 9.4)   (from table 9.4)

Female

Participant's name: _____

Date: _____/_____/_____

Circle the best trial:

Trial 1: _____ (in.)

Trial 2: _____ (in.)

Trial 3: _____ (in.)

Percentile: _____ Rating: _____
(from table 9.4)   (from table 9.4)

Thomas Test

Participant's name: _____ Date: _____/_____/_____

Right leg hip flexors: ☐ Flexible ☐ Inflexible

Left leg hip flexors: ☐ Flexible ☐ Inflexible

Straight-Leg-Raise Test

Participant's name: _____ Date: _____/_____/_____

Right leg hip extensors: ____° flexion ☐ Acceptable ☐ Unacceptable

Left leg hip extensors: ____° flexion ☐ Acceptable ☐ Unacceptable

From E. Acevedo and M. Starks, 2011, *Exercise testing and prescription lab manual*, 2nd ed. (Champaign, IL: Human Kinetics).

%HRR and %$\dot{V}O_2$R Calculation Worksheet

%HRR: (HRmax – Resting HR)
$\times$ % Intensity + Resting HR = Target HR

%$\dot{V}O_2$R: ($\dot{V}O_2$max – Resting $\dot{V}O_2$)
$\times$ % Intensity + Resting $\dot{V}O_2$= Target $\dot{V}O_2$

%HRR

_____ HRmax
– _____ Resting HR
= _____
$\times$ _____ % Intensity (50-80%)
= _____
+ _____ Resting HR
= _____ Target HR

%$\dot{V}O_2$R

_____ $\dot{V}O_2$max
– 3.5 ml/kg/min _____ Resting $\dot{V}O_2$
= _____
$\times$ _____ % Intensity (50-80%)
= _____
+ _____ Resting $\dot{V}O_2$
= _____ Target $\dot{V}O_2$

From E. Acevedo and M. Starks, 2011, *Exercise testing and prescription lab manual*, 2nd ed. (Champaign, IL: Human Kinetics).

Appendix C

Pharmacological Effects on Cardiorespiratory Responses to Exercise

Anticoagulant Agents

Category	Medication information	
Common drugs	*Generic name*	*Brand name*
	Heparin	Hepathrom, Lipo-hepin
	Warfarin	Coumadin
	Cilostazol	Pletal
	Clopidogrel	Plavix
	Dipyridamole	Persantine

Treatment	Thromboembolic conditions
	   1. Myocardial infarction
	   2. Rheumatic heart disease
	   3. Cerebrovascular disease	

Mechanism	Heparin inactivates thrombin and therefore prevents conversion of fibrinogen to fibrin. Coumadin inhibits synthesis of the vitamin K–dependent clotting factors.	
Adaptation for exercise Prescription	Does not seem to interfere with graded exercise testing.	

Anti-Anxiety Agents

Category	Medication Information	
Common drugs	*Generic name*	*Brand name*
	Meprobamate	Miltown, Equanil
	Chlordiazepoxide	Librium
	Diazepam	Valium
Treatment	Prescribe anti-anxiety agent.	
Mechanism	Varies.	
Effect at rest	Mild hypotension, no significant effects on hemodynamics or ECG findings, with exception of possible lowering of HR and BP	
Effect during exercise	No effect on exercise capacity	

Anti-Lipidemic Agents

Category	Medication information	
Common drugs	*Generic name*	*Brand name*
	Nicotinic Acid	Nicobid, Nicolar, Slo-Niacin, Niaspan
	Clofibrate	Artomid-S
	Cholestyrimine	Cuemid, Questram
	Probucol	Lorelco
	Colestipol	Colestid
	Gemfibrozil	Lopid

Category	Medication information	
Common drugs *(cont'd)*	*Generic name*	*Brand name*
	Atorvastatin	Lipitor
	Fluvastatin	Lescol
	Lovastatin	Mevacor
	Pravastatin	Pravachol
	Simvastatin	Zocor
	Ezetimibe	Zeta
Treatment	Reduction of elevated serum lipids to reduce morbidity and mortality in atherosclerosis and coronary artery disease.	
Mechanism	To reduce serum or plasma cholesterol.	
Effect at rest	With some exceptions, these agents have no effect on HR, BP, or ECG.	
Effect during exercise	These agents would not affect exercise tolerance in any direct fashion and would not interfere with graded exercise testing.	

Anti-Arrhythmic Agents

Category	Medication information	
Common drugs	*Generic name*	*Brand name*
	Digoxin	Lanoxin
	Diphenylhydantoin	Dilantin
	Lidocaine	Xylocaine
	Procainamide	Pronestyl
	Propranolol	Inderal
	Quinidine	Cardioquin
	Disopyramide	Norpace
	Verapamil	Isoptin
	Flecainide	Tambocor
	Propafenone	Rythmol
	Amiodarone	Cordarone, Pacerone
	Sotalol	Betapace
Treatment	To regulate abnormal cardiac rhythms.	
Mechanism	All anti-arrhythmics are used to normalize rhythm disturbances through diverse mechanisms. 1. Norpace: Decreases NA conductance, reduces conduction velocity 2. Dilantin: Increases K conductance, decreases conduction velocity and depressed NA conductance in ischemic tissues 3. Inderal: Produces beta-adrenergic receptor blockage 4. Isoptin: Blocks calcium channel activity	

(continued)

Anti-Arrhythmic Agents *(continued)*

Category	Medication information
Effect at rest	Reestablishes normal heart rhythm, which results in more efficient functioning, which results in reduced demand for oxygen; resting values can be varied.
Effect during exercise	By restoring a normal sinus rhythm, anti-arrhythmics improve exercise tolerance by allowing the heart to function more efficiently. Each of the classes of drugs will also modify the ECG.
Adaptation for exercise prescription	Exercise test for purpose of exercise prescription need not be performed because these agents do not significantly affect HR, but it is recommended that these drugs be used at time of test due to their effect on cardiac rhythm.

Beta-Blocking Agents

Category	Medication information	
Common drugs	*Generic name*	*Brand name*
	Acebutolol	Sectral
	Propranolol	Inderal
	Metoprolol	Lopressor
	Nadolol	Corgard
	Atenolol	Tenormin
	Pindolol	Visken
	Timilolol	Blocadren
	Sotalol	Betaspace
	Timolol	Blocadren
Treatment	Angina pectoris, hypertension, previous MI patients, arrhythmias, migraine headaches.	
Mechanism	Molecules of drug attach to beta-receptor sites of sympathetic nervous system throughout body, blocking catecholamines from attaching to sites. Some cardioselective agents act primarily on beta-2 receptors in the heart (relaxation of vascular and smooth muscle), whereas others have more agonist activity, stimulating rather than blocking receptors. (Beta-1 moderates cardiac stimulation.) Decreases heart's oxygen demands (myocardial oxygen consumption) and therefore workload by a slowing of the heart and decrease in contractility and blood pressure. May delay onset of the ischemic response.	
Effect at rest	Decreased HR, BP, and arrhythmias; pindolol does not affect resting hemodynamics.	
Effect during exercise	Increased exercise capacity in patients with angina, decreased exercise capacity in patients without angina, decreased exercise ischemia, decreased HR and BP; $\dot{V}O_2$max not affected.	
Adaptation for exercise prescription	Addition or withdrawal of beta-blocker to the therapeutic regimen of a patient necessitates a new graded exercise test. Relationship between %$\dot{V}O_2$R and %HRR is not altered; therefore, usual methods to calculate THR for exercise prescription are still acceptable. HRmax and training HR will be lower in persons receiving beta-blockers. Use HRmax with beta-blocker therapy.	

Broncodilators/Antihistamines

Category	Medication Information	
Common drugs	Generic name	Brand name
	Beclomethasone	Beclovent, Qvar
	Budesonide	Pulmicort
	Flunisolide	AeroBid
	Fluticasone	Flovent
	Albuterol	Proventil, Ventolin
	Metaproterenol	Alupent
	Salmeterol	Serevent
	Ipratropium	Atrovent
	Theophylline	Theo-Dur, Uniphyl
	Montelukast	Singulair
	Zileuton	Zyflo
	Cromolyn	Intal
	Omalizumab	Xolair
Treatment	Asthma, chronic obstructive pulmonary disease (COPD).	
Mechanism	Inhibit bronchial smooth-muscle constriction in patients with asthma or COPD.	
Effect at rest	May increase HR; may produce arrhythmia; BP effect will vary.	
Effect during exercise	May increase HR; may increase BP; may produce PVCs and dysrhythmias. Increases exercise capacity in patients limited by bronchospasms. Antihistamines: No effects on hemodynamic variables, the findings of resting or exercise ECG's, or exercise capacity.	

Calcium Channel Blockers

Category	Medication information	
Common drugs	Generic name	Brand name
	Verapamil	Isoptin, Calan
	Nifedipine	Procardia XL
	Diltiazem	Cardizem
Treatment	Angina pectoris, coronary artery spasm, arrhythmias, hypertension.	
Mechanism	Inhibits inward flow of calcium into cardiac and vascular smooth muscle, so calcium cannot pull troponin off actin to expose active site for crossbridge of myosin. Results in potent vasodilation, which increases coronary blood flow and supply and decreases slow-channel conductance of cardiac impulses. Affects strength of contraction.	
Effect at rest	Decreased HR (except for nifedipine/Procardia) and decreased BP.	
Effect during exercise	Same as rest; may increase exercise capacity. Normal ischemic response generally not blunted. Agents (except nifedipine) prolong the PR interval (delay the electrical conduction through the atrioventricular mode in the heart), with few other ECG effects.	

(continued)

Calcium Channel Blockers (continued)

Category	Medication information
Adaptation for exercise prescription	Addition or withdrawal of a calcium blocker to the therapeutic regimen of patient necessitates a new graded exercise test. Exercise prescription should be calculated by using data from an exercise test performed with the patient following the usual medical regimen.

Digitalis

Category	Medication information	
Common drugs	*Generic name*	*Brand name*
	Digoxin	Lanoxin
	Digitoxin	Crystodigin
	Digitalis	Digitortis
Treatment	Congestive heart failure (CHF), atrial fibrillation, atrial flutter.	
Mechanism	Improves myocardial contraction by altering the calcium utilization of the myocardial cell.	
Effect at rest	No significant change in HR, BP, or exercise capacity, except for a decrease in HR due to vagal effect.	
Effect during exercise	May decrease HR; will improve exercise capacity only in patients with atrial fibrillation or chronic heart failure (CHF). May produce false-positive results on the ECG, or ST segment depression in patients without coronary artery disease or ischemia. Use should be stopped 10 to 14 days prior to exercise test if possible.	

Diuretics

Category	Medication Information	
Common drugs	*Generic name*	*Brand name*
	Furosemide	Lasix, Furoside
	Triamterene	Dyazide
	Chlorothiazide	Diuril
	Spironolactone	Aldactone
	Amiloride	Midamor
Treatment	Hypertension, edema (swelling—cardiac, renal, hepatic).	
Mechanism	Most diuretics alter renal function, resulting in increased excretion of electrolytes and fluid by the following means: 1. Benzothiazides inhibit reabsorption of sodium and chloride in the distal tubule. 2. Loop diuretics inhibit sodium and chloride reabsorption in the ascending loop of Henle. 3. Potassium-sparing diuretics are antagonist of aldosterone, or inhibit sodium reabsorption and potassium excretion. Reduction of blood pressure and venous return in those with hypertension, reduced workload on heart, therefore, reduced O_2 demand.	
Effect at rest	No effect on HR; may decrease BP.	

Category	Medication Information
Effect during exercise	May decrease BP; may affect CHF patient, may induce arrhythmias (PVCs due to hypokalemia). HR or exercise capacity is typically not affected; however, hypovolemia may result in decreases in cardiac output, renal perfusion, and blood pressure.
Adaptation for exercise prescription	Check for hypokalemic conditions in patients receiving diuretics. Hypotension possible in postexercise period caused by hypovolemia; avoid dehydration before and after exercise; increase cool-down period.

Nitrates

Category	Medication information	
Common drugs	Generic name	Brand name
	Amyl nitrite	Amyl Nitrite
	Isosorbid mononitrate	Ismo, Imdur, Monoket
	Isosorbid dinitrate	Dilatrate, Isordil
	Nitroglycerin, sublingual, transligual, transmucosal, sustained release, transdermal, topical	Nitro-bid, Nitrostat, Nitrolingual, Nitrogard, Nitrong, Nitro-Dur, Nitrol
Treatment	Angina pectoris (used with beta-blocker or calcium channel blocker to reduce workload).	
Mechanism	Nitrates relax the smooth muscle of blood vessels by a direct effect, causing vasodilation. Decreased venous return causes decreased preload; arterial dilation decreases vascular resistance and arterial blood pressure.	
Effect at rest	Increased heart rate, decreased blood pressure, decreased workload and O_2 consumption of heart.	
Effect during exercise	Increased heart rate, decreased blood pressure, increased anginal threshold, increased exercise capacity, but decreased arterial pressure may result in hypotension.	
Adaptation for exercise prescription	Use of medication prior to reduce anginal occurrence. Longer for cool-down in postexercise period to reduce possibility of postural hypotension. Prescription involving target heart rate needs no alteration.	

Psychotropic Agents

Category	Medication Information	
Common drugs	Generic name	Brand name
	(major tranquilizer)	
	phenothiazine	Thorazine, Mellaril
Treatment	Prescribe antipsychotic medications, major tranquilizers.	
Mechanism	Anticholinergic and direct myocardial depressant alpha-adrenergic blockade.	
Effect at rest	May result in elevated HR, decreased BP, or orthostatic hypertension. The following ECG changes occur: increased PR and QT intervals (electrical conduction abnormalities), QRS widening, ST segment depression, blunting of T-wave.	

Sympatholytics (Drugs Interfering With SNS)

Category	Medication information	
Common drugs	*Generic name*	*Brand name*
	Reserpine	Serpasil
	Guanethidine	Ismelin
	Alpha-methyldopa	Aldomet
	Prazosin	Minipress
	Carvedilol	Coreg
Treatment	Treatment of hypertension.	
Mechanism	A variety of mechanisms exist, but all agents interfere with the effects of the SNS on the blood vessels or the heart by depleting or preventing the release of NE, reducing HR and contractility, decreasing activity of the SNS in the brain, or blocking alpha receptors in the vessels causing vasodilatation.	
Effect at rest	May decrease resting HR; decreases resting BP. Reserpine may cause depression, fatigue, and decreased desire for exercise.	
Effect during exercise	May decrease HR; decreases BP. No effect noted on ECG or exercise capacity.	
Adaptation for exercise prescription	Some medications may produce orthostatic hypotension, especially immediately after exercise. Gradual cool-down recommended.	

Tricyclic Antidepressants

Category	Medication Information	
Common drugs	*Generic name*	*Brand name*
	Imipramine, Amitriptyline	Tofranil, Elavil
	Desipramine	Norpramin
Treatment	Prescribe antidepressant.	
Mechanism	Block intake of NE in CNS.	
Effect at rest	May have increased HR, lower BP, increased tendency for arrhythmias, orthostatic hypotension, inversion or flattening of T-wave, possible false-positive test results.	

Vasodilators

Category	Medication information	
Common drugs	*Generic name*	*Brand name*
	Hydralazine	Apresoline
	Minoxidil	Loniten
	Captopril	Capoten
	Benazepril	Lotensin
	Ramipril	Altace
Treatment	Hypertension, CHF.	

Category	Medication information
Mechanism	Hydralazine and minoxidil act directly on vascular smooth muscle to cause relaxation and dilation. Captopril inhibits angiotensin-converting enzyme (ACE), which indirectly results in vasodilation (inhibits conversion of AI to vasoconstrictor AII). This vasodilation reduces blood pressure (decreases afterload). Results in decreased blood pressure and workload of the heart. Undesirable effects include increased HR and contractility, which impose a greater workload on the heart.
Effect at rest	Decrease in BP, possible increase in HR.
Effect during exercise	Reflex tachycardia, which may bring on anginal response. Postexercise hypotension may be accentuated by any of these medications.
Adaptation for exercise prescription	Gradual cool-down for prevention of hypotension after exercise. Effects of medications on exercise prescription are related to their effects on HR. Exercise prescription should be based on exercise test results while medicated.

Other Agents

Category	Medication Information
Alcohol	• Depresses heart indirectly by acting within the CNS. • Recent studies show chronic excessive use has a deleterious effect on the heart (may produce myocardial damage). • Not a coronary vasodilator. • Alcohol may prevent the sensation of anginal pain, probably due to central depressant effects. • Alcohol will not suppress the ECG changes that occur with exercise testing in patients with coronary atherosclerosis, but it may suppress associated anginal pain.
Thyroid medications	• When used to correct thyroid abnormality, and maintain state of euthyroidism, no abnormal cardiovascular effects. • Levothyroxine (Synthrox)—may produce elevations of HR and BP at rest and during exercise; cardiac arrhythmias, possible ischemia and angina.
Cold remedies	• Phenylpropanolamine, phenylephrine, pseudoephedrine • These agents may transiently increase HR and BP.

Nicotine	• Ganglionic stimulant causing vasoconstriction, elevated blood pressure, and tachycardia, resulting in increased cardiac workload .
	• Because of release of epinephrine and NE, resulting effects include increases in HR and SBP, DBP, and pulse pressures.
	• Excessive use may cause
	  - premature systole,
	  - atrial tachycardia,
	  - decrease in amplitude and inversion of T-wave, or
	  - angina and myocardial ischemia, atrial or ventricular arrhythmias.

Appendix D

Metric Conversions

Length Conversions

1 m = 39.370 in. = 3.281 ft = 1.0936 yd

1 cm = 0.3937 in.

1 mm = 0.03937 in.

1 km = 0.62137 mile

1 in. = 2.54 cm = 25.4 mm = 0.0254 m

1 ft = 0.3048 m

1 yd = 0.914 m = 91.44 cm

1 mile = 1609.35 m = 1.609 km

Mass (M) or Weight (Wt) Conversions

1 kg = 1 kp = 2.2046 lb

1 g = 0.0022 lb = 0.0352 oz

1 lb = 453.59 g = 0.454 kg

1 oz = 28.349 g

1 grain = 65 mg

Force (F) Conversions

1 kg = 9.80665 N

1 N = 0.10197 kg = 0.2248 lb

Volume (V) Conversions

1 L = 1.0567 US qt (1 US qt and 1 US gal are >1 Imperial qt and gal)

1 US qt = 0.9464 L

1 US gal = 3.785 L

1 cup liquid = 250 ml

1 tablespoon = 15 ml

Work (w) and Energy (E) Conversions

1 Nm = 1 J = 0.7375 ft-lb

1 kgm = 9.80665 J = 7.2307 ft-lb

1 ft-lb = 0.1383 kgm = 1.3560 Nm

1 kJ = 0.239 kcal

1 kcal = 4186 J = 4.186 kJ

1 kcal = 426.85 kgm at 100% efficiency

1 J = 0.10197 kgm

1 liter of oxygen used in burning glycogen (respiratory quotient = 1.0)

= 5.0047 kcal

= 15,575 ft-lb

= 2153 kgm $\cdot$ min^{-1}

Velocity (v) Conversions

1 m $\cdot$ s^{-1} = 2.2371 mph

1 m $\cdot$ min^{-1} = 0.03728 mph

1 km $\cdot$ h^{-1} (kmh) = 0.6215 mph

1 mph = 26.8 m $\cdot$ min^{-1}

Radial Velocity Conversions

1 rad $\cdot$ s^{-1} = 57.3° $\cdot$ s^{-1}

rad = radian = 0.5 π = radius of circle = 57.3°

1° = 0.01745 radian

π = 3.1416 = ratio of the circumference of a circle to its diameter

Power (P) Conversions

1 W = 1 J $\cdot$ s^{-1} = 60 J $\cdot$ min^{-1} = 0.060 kJ $\cdot$ min^{-1} = 6.12 kgm $\cdot$ min^{-1}
= 0.1019 kgm $\cdot$ s^{-1}

1 kW = 1000 W = 1.34 hp

1 kgm $\cdot$ min^{-1} = 0.1635 W = 0.000219 hp

1 hp = 745.7 W = 745.7 J $\cdot$ s^{-1} = 75 kgm $\cdot$ s^{-1} = 4562 kgm $\cdot$ min^{-1}
= 10.688 kcal $\cdot$ min^{-1}

Acceleration (a) Conversion

a of gravity = 9.81 m $\cdot$ s^2 = 32.2 ft $\cdot$ s^2

Temperature (T) Conversions

each °C = 1 °K = 1.8 °F

each °F = 0.56 °C = 0.56 °K

Pressure Units, Symbols, and Conversions

1 Pascal (Pa) = 1 N $\cdot$ m^2

Barometric pressure (PB): 1 in. = 25.4 torr; 29.92 in. Hg = 760 torr
= 1 atm = 14.7 lb/in.

1 mbar = 0.750 mm Hg = 0.750 torr

Appendix E

Metabolic and Anthropometric Equations

Metabolic Equations

Walking

This formula is suitable for speeds of 50 to 100 m/min (1.9 to 3.7 mph).

$$\dot{V}O_2 = 0.1 \text{ (speed)} + 1.8 \text{ (speed)(fractional grade)} + 3.5 \text{ ml/kg/min}$$

Running

This formula is suitable for speeds of 80 to over 134 m/min (3.0 to 5.0 mph) if the participant is jogging or running.

$$\dot{V}O_2 = 0.2 \text{ (speed)} + 0.9 \text{ (speed)(fractional grade)} + 3.5 \text{ ml/kg/min}$$

Leg Ergometry

These formulas are suitable for power outputs between 50 and 200 Watts (300 – 1,200 kg/m/min).

$$\dot{V}O_2 = 1.8 \text{ (work rate)} \bullet M^{-1} + 7 \text{ ml/kg/min}$$

or

$$\dot{V}O_2 = \frac{1.8 \text{ (work rate)}}{M} + 7 \text{ ml/kg/min}$$

Arm Ergometry

These formulas are suitable for power outputs between 25 and 125 Watts (150-750 kg/m/min).

$$\dot{V}O_2 = 3 \text{ (work rate)} M^{-1} + 3.5 \text{ ml/kg/min}$$

or

$$\dot{V}O_2 = \frac{3 \text{ (work rate)}}{M} + 3.5 \text{ ml/kg/min}$$

Stepping

This formula is suitable for stepping rates between 12 and 30 steps/min, and step height between 0.04 and 0.40 m (1.6-15.7 in.).

$$\dot{V}O_2 = 0.2 \text{ (stepping rate)} + 1.33 \bullet 1.8 \text{ (step height) (stepping rate)} + 3.5 \text{ ml/kg/min}$$

Anthropometric Equations

Skinfold Formulas for Determining Body Density

Jackson-Pollock 7-site formula for men (chest, midaxillary, triceps, subscapular, abdomen, suprailiac, and thigh):

Body density = 1.112 – 0.00043499 (sum of 7 skinfolds)
+ 0.00000055 (sum of 7 skinfolds)^2 – 0.00028826 (age)

Jackson-Pollock 3-site formula for men (chest, abdomen, and thigh):

Body density = 1.10938 – 0.0008267 (sum of 3 skinfolds)
+ 0.0000016 (sum of 3 skinfolds)^2 – 0.0002574 (age)

Jackson-Pollock 3-site formula for men (chest, triceps, and subscapular):

Body density = 1.1125025 – 0.0013125 (sum of 3 skinfolds)
+ 0.0000055 (sum of 3 skinfolds)^2 – 0.000244 (age)

Jackson-Pollock 7-site formula for women (chest, midaxillary, triceps, subscapular, abdomen, suprailiac, and thigh):

Body density = 1.097 – 0.00046971 (sum of 7 skinfolds)
+ 0.00000056 (sum of 7 skinfolds)^2 – 0.00012828 (age)

Jackson-Pollock 3-site formula for women (triceps, suprailiac, and thigh):

Body density = 1.099421 – 0.0009929 (sum of 3 skinfolds)
+ 0.0000023 (sum of 3 skinfolds)^2 – 0.0001392 (age)

Jackson/Pollock 3-site formula for women (triceps, suprailiac, and abdomen):

Body density = 1.089733 – 0.0009245 (sum of 3 skinfolds)
+ 0.0000025 (sum of 3 skinfolds)^2 – 0.0000979 (age)

Body Density to Body Fat Conversion Formulas

Brozek body density conversion formula:

$$\frac{457}{\text{body density}} - 414.2 = \%\text{body fat}$$

Siri body density conversion formula:

$$\frac{495}{\text{body density}} - 450 = \%\text{body fat}$$

Determining Goal Body Fat Percentage and Target Weight

The following method can be used to determine goal body fat percentage (GBF%) and target weight (TW):

1. Multiply total body weight (TBW) by the body fat percentage (BF%) to determine fat weight (FW).
2. Subtract FW from TBW.
3. The remaining weight is the lean mass weight (LMW).
4. Determine an appropriate and reasonable GBF%.
5. Divide the LMW by the GBF% − 1.
6. The answer will be the TW at the predetermined GBF%.
7. Subtract TW from TBW to determine the amount of weight loss (WL) required to achieve GBF%.

Step-by-step instructions are as follows:

Step 1	TBW × BF% = FW
Step 2	TBW − FW = LMW
Step 3	LMW/(GBF% − 1) = TW
Step 4	TBW − TW = WL

Appendix F

Lab 11 Answer Key

Problem 1
  a. 46.18 ml/kg/min
  b. 3.69 L/min
  c. 13.2 METs
  d. 18.45 kcal/min
  e. 830.25 total kcal

Problem 2
  a. 40 ml/kg/min
  b. 3.31 L/min
  c. 11.43 METs
  d. 16.55 kcal/min
  e. 622 total kcal

Problem 3
  a. 27.06 ml/kg/min
  b. 7.73 METs
  c. 8% grade
  d. 11.5 kcal/min
  e. 345 total kcal

Problem 4
  a. 36.79 ml/kg/min
  b. 2.1 L/min
  c. 10.5 METs
  d. 10.5 kcal/min
  e. 313.5 total kcal

Problem 5
  a. 32.73 ml/kg/min
  b. 2.9 L/min
  c. 9.3 METs
  d. 14.5 kcal/min
  e. 652.5 total kcal

Problem 6
  a. 23.86 ml/kg/min
  b. 1.3 L/min
  c. 6.8 METs
  d. 6.4 kcal/min
  e. 192 total kcal

Problem 7
  a. 53.03 ml/kg/min
  b. 4.1 L/min
  c. 15.2 METs
  d. 20.5 kcal/min
  e. 40.65 ml/kg/min

Problem 8
  a. 5.5 kcal/min
  b. 330 total kcal
  c. 19.52 ml/kg/min
  d. 5.6 METs
  e. 3.4% grade

Problem 9
  a. 19.21 ml/kg/min
  b. 1.1 L/min
  c. 5.5 METs
  d. 5.5 kcal
  e. 16.07 ml/kg/min

Problem 10
  a. 4.36 L/min
  b. 6.27 mph
  c. 12.7 METs
  d. 22 kcal/min
  e. 660 total kcal

From E. Acevedo and M. Starks, 2011, *Exercise testing and prescription lab manual*, 2nd ed. (Champaign, IL: Human Kinetics).

Glossary

aneurysm—A bulging of the wall of a blood vessel, usually caused by hardening of the arteries and high blood pressure.

angina—A symptom of some diseases that is characterized by a feeling of choking, suffocation, or crushing pressure and pain.

artifact—A distortion that does not reflect a true waveform found within electrocardiography. Often caused by excessive lead wire motion or improper electrode placement.

body composition—The percentage of body weight that is fat (% body fat) compared to total lean mass.

Chatillon scale—A hanging weight scale.

claudication—Pain of the legs consisting of cramps in the calves caused by poor circulation of blood in the legs.

dynamometer—An instrument that operates on the compression principle and is used to indicate the force required to move a needle a certain distance.

electrocardiograph—A device that records the electric activity of the heart to detect abnormal electric impulses through the muscle.

electrocardiogram (ECG)—An electrical record of the current flowing through the heart muscle during the depolarization and repolarization of a contraction.

embolism—A defect in which a clot (embolus) travels through the bloodstream and becomes lodged in a blood vessel, usually in the heart, lungs, or brain.

ergometer—An instrument used to measure the amount of work done by an organism.

ergometry—A method of measuring the amount of work done by an organism, usually during exertion.

flexibility—The ability to move the body parts through a wide range of motion.

goniometer—A protractor type of instrument used to measure the total degrees of rotation of a joint.

Gulick tape—A flexible measuring tape equipped with a spring-loaded attachment at the end that, when pulled out to a specified mark, exerts a fixed amount of tension on the tape.

isokinetic training—Training that has both variable resistance and a speed-governing feature. Because isokinetic equipment controls the rate of contraction, it can potentially train the different types of muscle fibers.

isometric contraction—A static muscle contraction wherein the overall length of the muscle does not change during the application of force against a fixed object.

isotonic contraction—A dynamic muscle contraction in which the force remains constant. Isotonic exercises are typically performed with free weights or machines in which the resistance is steered along a fixed path. Accommodating resistance training (e.g., Nautilus, Cybex, etc.) is considered isotonic, although resistance is variable so that the lifter must exert maximum effort throughout the full range of motion.

Korotkoff—Five phases of varying sounds heard through auscultation during blood pressure assessment.

linearity—The maximum percentage of error between the expected value and the actual sensor reading, throughout an instrument's measurement range.

maximal oxygen consumption—The highest amount of oxygen a person can take in and utilize to produce adenosine triphosphate aerobically during heavy exercise.

moderate exercise—Activities that are approximately 3 to 6 metabolic equivalents (METs) or the equivalent of brisk walking at 3 to 4 mph for most healthy adults.

muscular endurance—The ability of a muscle to exert a submaximal force over a length of time.

muscular strength—The maximum amount of force that a muscle can exert in a single maximal effort.

one-repetition maximum (1RM)—The maximum weight that a person can lift successfully for one repetition.

open-circuit spirometry—A method for estimating oxygen consumption in which the subject breathes in air directly from the atmosphere. The composition of the air is measured as it flows in and out of the lungs.

principle of overload—repeated exposure, including appropriate rest, to unaccustomed load is associated with adaptation of improved functional capacity

principle of specificity—specific adaptations from specific stimulus to specific systems involved

principle of progression—improved functioning requires increases in stimulus to cause further adaptation.

random error—An error that is a result of pure chance.

reliability—the extent to which your assessment yields the same result on repeated trials.

scale—An instrument used to measure gross body weight.

skinfold calipers—A pincher device that measures the thickness of a double layer of finger-pinched skin and subcutaneous fat.

specificity of training—the training stimulus should be relevant and appropriate to the adaptation for which the individual is training in order to produce a training effect.

sphygmomanometer—An instrument made up of a rubber bladder, gauge, and rubber inflation/deflation bulb and valve that is used to measure systolic and diastolic blood pressure.

stadiometer—An instrument used to measure standing height.

stethoscope—An instrument made up of an amplification bell, a Y-shaped rubber tubing, and earpieces used to detect sounds produced by the human body.

systematic error—A predictable error systematically influenced by something other than what you are attempting to measure.

validity—the accuracy of your assessment; whether or not you are assessing what you have intended to assess.

Valsalva maneuver—Increased pressure in the abdominal and thoracic cavities caused by breath holding and extreme effort. Performing a Valsalva maneuver can inhibit the return of blood to the heart and increase blood pressure.

vigorous exercise—Activities of greater that 6 METs or, alternatively, an exercise intense enough to represent a substantial cardiorespiratory challenge. If a person's exercise capacity is known, vigorous exercise may be defined as an intensity of greater than 60% maximum oxygen uptake.

$\dot{V}O_2$—The rate at which oxygen is being transported to and used by the active working tissues of the body.

$\dot{V}O_2$**max**—The maximal rate at which oxygen can be transported to and used by the working tissues of the body. The most accepted index of cardiorespiratory work.

$\dot{V}O_2$**peak**—the highest $\dot{V}O_2$ achieved during a max test. Often this term describes $\dot{V}O_2$ when the criterion for $\dot{V}O_2$max is not met.

$\dot{V}O_2$**reserve ($\dot{V}O_2$R)**—The difference between $\dot{V}O_2$max and resting $\dot{V}O_2$.

About the Authors

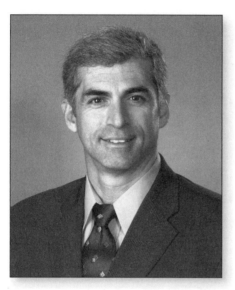

Edmund O. Acevedo, PhD, is a professor and chair of the department of health and human performance at Virginia Commonwealth University.

He is a fellow of the American College of Sports Medicine and the American Psychological Association. He is an ACSM-certified clinical exercise specialist. His 21-year career in research and teaching has cemented his commitment to standardized fundamentals for exercise testing and prescription.

Dr. Acevedo makes his home in Midlothian, Virginia, with his wife, Tracy, and their two children. In his free time, he enjoys on- and off-road running and biking.

Michael A. Starks, PhD, is an adjunct professor in the college of counseling, educational psychology, and research at the University of Memphis.

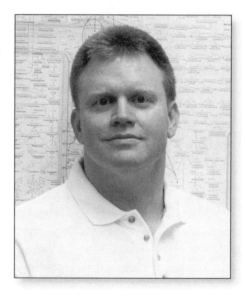

He is a certified strength and conditioning specialist from the National Strength and Conditioning Association and is a CPR and first aid instructor for the National Safety Council and American Red Cross.

Starks makes his home in Germantown, Tennessee, with his wife, Stacy, and three children. In his free time, he enjoys resistance training, competing in triathlons, and coaching.

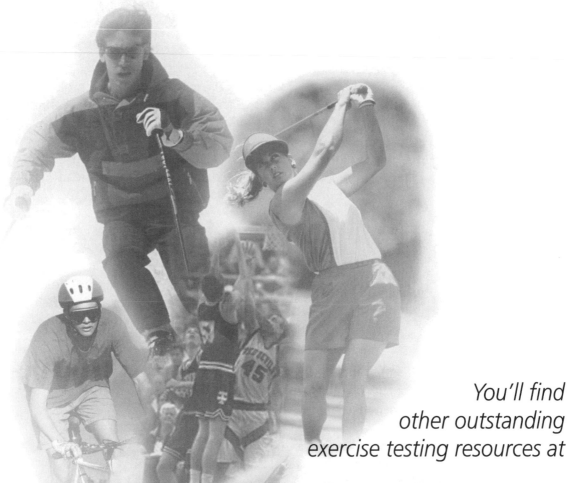